VAST INSTITUTE

KINDLING THE FLAME

THE ART AND SCIENCE OF COGNITIVE REPLENISHMENT

9/20/21

*Debbie, we
may you emagene
a better world into
being, with ease + joy.*

*warmest
Michelle*

Kindling the Flame

The Art and Science of Cognitive Replenishment

Michelle Sherman

Founder of the VAST Institute®

TABLE OF CONTENTS

FOREWORD

It is said that when the student is ready, the teacher will appear. I must have been ready when I met Michelle Sherman fifteen-years ago, although I would have described myself at that time more as lost and confused. I had left my homeland of Germany and a promising career in cardiology to venture off into the world of medical science. A PhD in molecular biology and several successful research projects later, I found myself once again stuck in a career that didn't fulfill me. This is when a friend pointed me towards Michelle and the Vast Institute. Following my friend's recommendation turned out to be one of the best decisions I've made in my life.

Michelle's skillful guidance and coaching were instrumental for me to discover my path and purpose. Even more importantly, I discovered aspects of myself I was previously unware of. With a powerful and unique mixture of clarity, humor, compassion and a staunch belief in my potential, Michelle was able lead me out of the pit of confusion and self-doubt. Through our work together I discovered my true passion, which is to help people to address and heal their emotional and physical challenges on subconscious, root-cause level.

Since then I have created a breakthrough program, which has helped thousands of people world-wide to overcome anxiety and depression, and wrote an award-winning book, The Fear and Anxiety Solution. Michelle's masterful coaching processes allowed me to recognize, unblock and bring to light the gifts and talents I am here to share with world. And for this I will be eternally grateful for her.

Her new book, *Kindling the Flame: the Art and Science of Cognitive Replenishment*, which is written with the same spirit of lightness, intelligence, kindness and depth I appreciated so much during our sessions, is timely and needed. The demands on our minds are exponentially greater than just a few decades ago. The enormous daily pressures, expectations and unprecedented amount of information we are exposed to, are the major reasons why stress, anxiety and depression became the number one health concern in most modern societies. With *Kindling the Flame* Michelle provides solid, research-based explanations on how we deplete our mental, emotional and creative capacities, and offers effective and enjoyable processes and tools to nourish and expand our mind to its optimal functioning.

Cognitive Replenishment is a gift for anyone who yearns to boost themselves to a higher level of joy, purpose, harmony and fulfillment. I am thrilled that with this book Michelle is sharing her wisdom and gifts with a world-wide audience. And I am certain that it will be a catalyst of healing and growth for its readers – just like Michelle has been for me.

–Dr. Friedemann Schaub, MD. PhD.

www.thefearandanxietysolution.com

CHAPTER ONE
Small Changes Made with Great Enthusiasm...

> *"The mind is not a vessel to be filled, but a fire to*
> *be kindled." –Plutarch, 66 A.D.*

Welcome to the VAST Institute® Cognitive Replenishment program.

Our goal is to offer a simple set of tools to mentally recharge your life. During this program you will learn how to intentionally kindle your flame, contributing to a healthier, more focused mind.

At the VAST Institute we wholeheartedly believe that you can significantly enhance your sense of well-being and quality of life by:

1. Intentionally nourishing your mind

2. Igniting a positive imagination

3. Taking command of where you focus your attention

4. Setting healthier boundaries

With these four techniques you will acquire the coveted treasure of a replenished mind.

A replenished mind flaunts itself in our day-to-day world by sharing ideas that inspire brilliant solutions. It ventures into unchartered territory with friends or colleagues. It creates new inventions, social movements or business solutions from the ether. Replenished minds positively impact relationships and ultimately society at large.

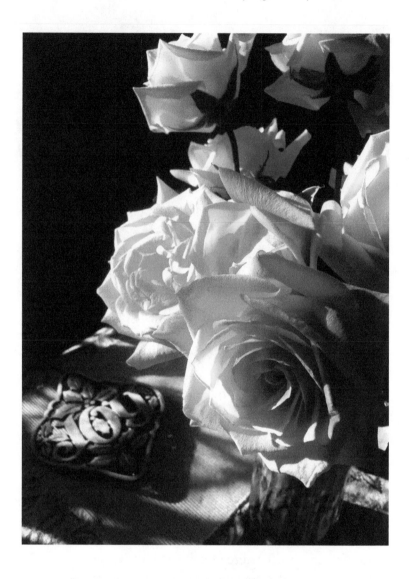

A refreshed mind has the capacity to instigate acts of kindness. It possesses a mental stamina that can imagine the essential goodness of humanity as the wellspring for right-action.

Cognitive Replenishment prepares you to engage your

positive imagination. As illustrated by scientific research, when we replenish our cognitive realm the systems and chemicals in our brains that kindle positive imagination more easily flow.

Exhibiting a positive imagination is an intentional and brave choice.

With a positive imagination you become a trendsetter, formulating unique solutions before those around you. Your imagination provides the placeholder for a brighter future until that future can actually occur.

One former client told me that by developing the Cognitive Replenishment practice I had "created one of the most effective and at the same time fun approaches to assist people in discovering and creating the life they may have never dared dream of." – F.S.

A Cognitive Replenishment practice enhances your unique brand of genius, and as a result enhances your contribution to work, community, or beloved family. The Middle English word "plenish" is derived from the Latin word plenus and means, "to fill up, stock or furnish".

Cognitive Replenishment is your admission ticket to Original Thinking. With Original Thinking in your pocket, you can engage with life in a manner that honors, nourishes and supports your best interests.

This VAST Institute course shares that which I have found personally effective, as well as with clients who were seeking to fully embody their greatness.

Anything ever created by humans was first conceived within their imagination. What would your life be like if you could imagine a path towards health, joy and greatness? What if the ability to work from a replenished mind is what a renowned thinker like Albert Einstein meant when he said, "We cannot solve our problems at the same level of thinking that created them"?

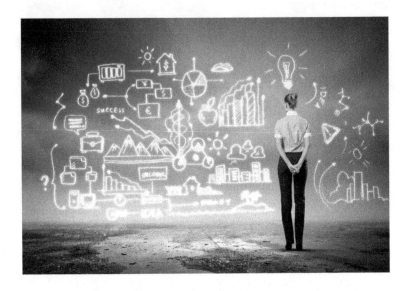

As a lifelong optimist with worryholic tendencies, I can personally attest to the healing benefits of an intentional Cognitive Replenishment practice. Over the past several years, with patience and good humor, I have transitioned from being a worryholic eighty-percent of the time to being a practical optimist eighty-percent of the time. I believe that I have made great progress within this lifetime.

Many of my clients feel similar, "Michelle has equipped me to face life with equanimity and enthusiasm. A clear assessment of any situation and related emotions leads to much better results than frantic worrying." – M.B.

Pick and choose the techniques or ideas that work best for you. Experiment with them. Small changes, when done with enthusiasm, can bring about satisfying results.

By the time you have completed this program you will be more comfortable as a practical optimist and will see how a simple Cognitive Replenishment practice can improve the quality of your life in real time.

If in reviewing this material you discover the need for deeper emotional support, please reach out to a trusted friend, mental health care professional, or a kindhearted spiritual advisor.

Cognitive exhaustion can wear us down. Its impact is real and can point even the best of us towards a bleaker perspective of the landscape. Each human being walking this planet has experienced moments of negativity. Please remember that many ills can be eased when we decide to make positive changes (such as those recommended in this book), and spend time in the company of those who genuinely care about our wellbeing.

With the VAST method you will learn to navigate the information rapids of modern life while staying alert, refreshed and relatively dry.

Practice your favorite VAST Cognitive Replenishment technique to revitalize your mind, strengthen your optimism and in the long run improve your view of the world. Tune-in to the ideas presented. Experiment with this opportunity to practice a few new "mind moves" in a safe and supportive environment. This set of life skills was designed to kindle your mind and inspire you to notice all that is already good in your world.

Sometimes taking on a Cognitive Replenishment practice means we get much more than we bargained for. "I didn't seek Michelle for personal counseling. What I came for and what I got surprised me. My relationship with my husband improved and keeps getting better. I was given a new way of thinking, sometimes radically different from my own…My attitude towards my life and my business has changed… My business is not my life." – C.E.

Your cognitive realm is a precious resource to be better understood and enjoyed. This primer is intended to harness that power on your own behalf and encourage you to share your contributions with the world at large. Uplift yourself as you help the world.

Ready?

Let us begin by imagining that the few simple concepts in this book can support you in crafting a more fulfilling life.

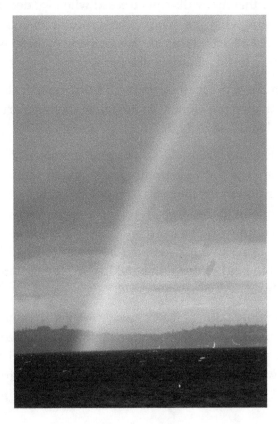

CHAPTER ONE
REVIEW QUESTIONS TO CONSIDER:

1. What does the *plenish* in cognitive replenishment mean?
2. Name two cognitive replenishment techniques.
3. What is the opposite of cognitive replenishment?
4. Why is developing a positive imagination worthwhile?
5. Name two benefits you stand to gain from a cognitive replenishment practice.

Cognition - the mental action or process of acquiring knowledge and understanding through thought, experience, and the senses.

Cognitive replenishment -

"and" thinking - allows for the optimistic explanation of a situation

CHAPTER TWO
Listen to Albert

Albert Einstein had two insights that inform and shape the VAST Institute® Cognitive Replenishment Practice:

1. "Imagination is more important than knowledge."

2. "We cannot solve our problems at the same level of thinking that created them."

Why did one of the greatest minds of our time believe that imagination trumps knowledge and that we require a new way of thinking to solve our seemingly insurmountable problems? It is because he understood that if we implement these two key ingredients we can amplify the quality of life for all who dwell on this planet.

You are the opportunity for wonderful things to be imagined and created. Through your choices you inspire others to think in ways that exemplify nobler instincts. Positive imagination is a fundamental element in achieving more harmonious outcomes both in our lives and the world at large.

If this is so, then why does the world often feel so out of balance? Why do we get caught up in our baser instincts when solving the problems that plague us?

What I discovered while coaching really bright and loving people over the years is simple: most people possess a good heart and the intelligence to be effective. However, their cognitive reserves are often quite depleted, diminishing their ability to tap into the creative force of their positive imagination. Their flame is dwindling and no longer fuels them. Thus the benefit of a Cognitive Replenishment practice is evident.

"I was too numb to acknowledge the supposed 'successes' I had attained... I was stressed and unhappy... I realized 'joy' was a long lost concept for me... Now I am *identifying* and *feeling* excitement and joy again, and creating a much healthier life for myself and my family." – W.L.G.

A positive imagination can range from powerful for some, to non-existent for others. If as children we were taught the set of mental skills that encourage our ability to envision a worthwhile future, we are ahead of the game. If we were never encouraged to develop optimism, we can feel frustrated and doubt the possibility of positive outcomes. None of us want to feel that disappointment again.

Belief in the sanctity of goodness can be ripped away from us before we are old enough to fight back if we have experienced abuse or neglect. Those who stay committed to a kindhearted approach to life are often portrayed as unrealistic, absurd, inconsequential, or weak. But this is far from true.

Then there are those of us who fall in to the highly sensitive range.

In her groundbreaking book, *Highly Sensitive People*, Elaine Aron, Ph.D., explains how approximately twenty-percent of most species are highly sensitive to stimulation. They are more easily over-aroused, becoming uncomfortable and shy as a result. Their sensitivity to all types of physical, emotional or energetic stimulation allows them to serve humanity as "the priest-judge-advisor class". She describes highly sensitive people as "a more thoughtful group, often checking the impulses of the warrior-kings. Since the advisor class often proves right, its members are respected

11

as counselors, historians, teachers, scholars, and the upholders of justice... They warn against hasty wars and bad use of land" (Aron, 1996, pg. 18).

Highly sensitive people possess a special type of personal power, which is not always appreciated.

"People who are gifted and intuitive yet conscientious and determined not to make mistakes ought to be treasured employees. But [highly sensitive people] are less likely to fit into the business world when the metaphors for achievement are warfare, pioneering and expansion." (Aron, 1996, pg. 128)

At VAST we believe that true power need not prove itself or abuse others. It does not need to. It already knows its worth.

For the highly sensitive and those who prefer to experience personal coherence, there is a wiser, gentler way to become more resilient in this world (McCraty, 2003). This is made possible through the practice of Cognitive Replenishment. Perhaps, as Albert suggested, imagining it first opens the path for it to be possible.

CHAPTER TWO
REVIEW QUESTIONS TO CONSIDER:

1. What does Albert think is more important than knowledge?

2. Name one reason people often lack a positive imagination.

3. Name one quality Highly Sensitive People (HSP) possess.

CHAPTER THREE

Why Does Our Inner "Negative Nellie" Often Steal the Show?

> *"The human mind is a channel through which things-to-be are coming into the realm of things-that-are." –Henry Ford, 1930*

All that we create individually or as a species begins with an idea, thought, or mental image. We each possess both positive and negative imagination, but unfortunately it often defaults to the negative. Here are two reasons why "Negative Nellie" steals the show, even when we wish it were otherwise.

First, we need to acknowledge the daily onslaught of negative messaging that inundates our lives without our full awareness or permission. Bad news arrives on our doorstep by newspaper, cyberspace and text message, unquestioned and unabated, spreading concerns that get our attention. "The world is a dangerous place"; "Every woman secretly wants to be a size four"; "Until you're a certain age no one will take you seriously"; " When you are beyond a certain age no one will take you seriously"; "The end justifies the means"; "It is impossible to trust *those people*"; "The nice guy finishes last"; "There were ten murders in your city last week"; "Schoolgirls halfway around the world are kidnapped by terrorists"; "Every man needs Viagra", etc., etc., etc. Furthermore, as we will discuss later, there is the subtle influence of those around us who would prefer for us to join them in their negative thought cycles. We've all heard the old saying, "misery loves company".

When repeatedly hearing messages that display the world in a fearsome manner, the subconscious mind soaks it up and focuses on the negative information exclusively, ignoring any positive evidence to the contrary. This is the result of a neurologically driven survival strategy that intentionally emphasizes bad news. We witness this in people who focus on one negative message while ignoring ten positives ones. Perhaps you can relate?

Sources of cognitive depletion in your life often go unnoticed. Graphic depictions of violence and messages of illness pervade our culture, inextricably embedded in myriad forms of entertainment. Violence promotes feelings of elation in some people due to a hard-wired adrenal response. Others become ill if they witness carnage and harm inflicted upon living creatures. Our nervous system reacts identically in response to real or portrayed violence.

this is why violin/violent students work. the brain sees it as the same whether real or "visioned"

Dennis Waitley, the renowned sports psychologist, explained that when they measured brain activity in athletes during Olympic training they discovered that practicing in their minds stimulated identical parts of the brain as actual physical activity did. Mental practice puts our brain through the regimen without the danger. This is just one sociobiological and practical use of the positive imagination (Waitley, 2010).

Illness messaging can also be erosive. Listening to potential side effects listed in pharmaceutical ads informs us of the risks of the medication, but also brings the thought of that pain and suffering into our living room. Those messages are introduced into your subconscious repeatedly.

This fuels thoughts of illness and horrid drug-induced side effects that you never even knew existed. Really? What is restless leg syndrome? Soon your negative imagination

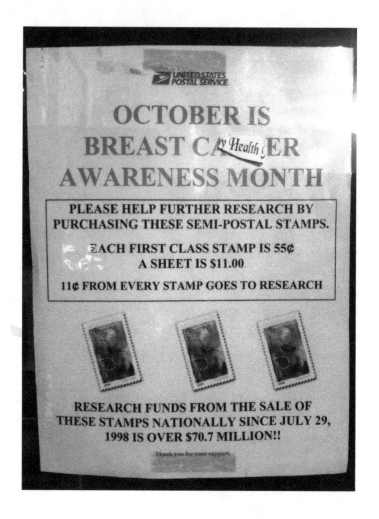

starts to focus on it. What if I have that disease? What if it's fatal? What if there is no cure? It's not healthy to be incessantly reminded of illness.

In addition, there is the onslaught of subliminal messages we are subjected to each day, both online and in real life. The Cambridge dictionary defines a "subliminal message" as: "Not recognized or understood by the conscious mind, but still having an influence on it:

Imperceptible or below the threshold of the conscious mind."

Where you direct your attention has an impact on situations. This is illustrated by the Hawthorne Effect, which states that an observer will unintentionally become part of the experiment and influences its results. What we focus on tends to magnify. So it is crucial to focus on what we want, instead of what we *do not* want.

Have you ever purchased a "Save Vanishing Species" or "Breast Cancer Awareness" stamp? You can buy them at the post office for a few cents over the current postal rate and all proceeds are donated to wildlife preservation and breast cancer awareness respectively.

I am quite touched by the commitment many have made to preserving species diversity and curing breast cancer ASAP. One of the most cost effective things I suggest we do is to rename those campaigns to reflect the desired outcome. I prefer to purchase stamps advocating for *species preservation and diversity* or *breast health*.

To address this unintentional negative message campaign, I wrote a letter to the US Postmaster General respectfully requesting we change the "Breast Cancer" stamp to the "Breast Health" stamp. It would benefit women more by having them focus on breast health in the pursuit of preventing and defeating cancer. I do not want to unintentionally spread the meme of breast cancer each time one of those stamps is purchased, seen, received or read. When I purchase the stamps I literally cross out the word "cancer" and write the word "health" above it. Someone actually amended this sign in the post office.

The world is often portrayed through a lens of sickness, cruelty, mistrust and destruction. This prism impacts our overall sense of wellbeing, so when we feel down, depressed, tired, frightened, hopeless, cynical, anxious, or mentally exhausted, we may not fully understand why. We may be unintentionally soaking up a negative worldview. If unchecked, these negative messages can result in chronic stress and exhaustion.

A study conducted after the Boston Marathon bombing, by the *National Academy of Science,* revealed that people in the U.S. exposed to more than six-hours-a-day of post marathon bombing media coverage, were nine-times more likely to report acute stress symptoms than people who experienced the bombing firsthand (National Academy of Science, 2013). Nine-times! The authors surmise that repeated exposure to violent images or sounds keep traumatic events alive longer and trigger physical fear and threat responses. Continuous response to a perceived threat can have serious health consequences over time, as discussed in further detail in chapter five.

Furthermore, the reason we default to our negative imagination is due to a survival mechanism wired into our brain and central nervous system. Humans are wired to respond to fear-based messages more vigorously than positive ones. This adaptation insures that we will notice any "bad news" that might prove to become life threatening. This is referred to as an amygdala hijack by Daniel Goleman in his seminal book, *Emotional Intelligence* (1997).

An amygdala hijack focuses our attention on problems instead of the solutions. Accordingly, countless inspiring and uplifting ideas, or examples of human kindness go unnoticed. We are less aware of the warm shower, food on the table, or neighbor generously helping neighbor. Our narrative is filtered through the emotional negativity demanded by the amygdala.

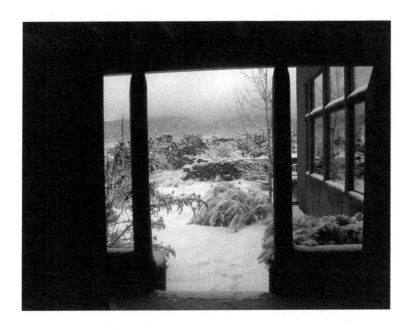

In June of 2014, a paper published by the National Academy of Science revealed that Facebook, Cornell University and the UC in San Francisco had collaborated in an online experiment involving 70,000 Facebook users. The goal was to determine the impact that filtering positive and negative messaging had on a Facebook users' emotional state. Although there is a question whether these customers gave informed consent, the findings are clear. Through intentional manipulation of news feeds, which provided positive, sad or angry words, Facebook provoked positive or negative feelings in their users. The outcome was that happy news feeds triggered happiness while sad news feeds triggered sadness without customer awareness of this manipulation (National Academy of Science, 2014).

Allowing our focus to incessantly dwell on what is wrong with this world can deplete us emotionally and compromise our health, as chronic stress is apt to do.

What we pay attention to, whether consciously or unconsciously, affects our emotional state and experience of life. The emotionally charged fear, sadness or anger of others that invades our space can shift our mood, erode our self-confidence and diminish our optimism.

> "Before I met [Michelle], I had a terrible time. I could not imagine anything good coming to me... You helped me clarify my life's purpose, and you gently guided me in creative, new, empowering beliefs and behaviors. I changed the way I react to negative situations and am much more effective at handling them. I now have a clear vision of how I will serve the world the rest of my life, a plan to make my dream real, and the conviction that I can make it happen."
> – D.E.

This emotional contagion occurs due to the presence of specific neurons in our brain that mirror the emotional state of those we spend time with, whether it is for peaceful assembly or to enact revenge. We do not always understand that who, and what, we expose ourselves to on a daily basis may fuel the sense of fear, sadness, shame or doom we are experiencing. We can mistakenly incorporate the pessimism of others as our reality, when those negative feelings may actually be the result of emotional contagion.

Rachel Dracht on Saturday Night Live brilliantly captured the essence of the "Negative Nellie" archetype in her portrayal of Debbie Downer, a woman who continually finds the dark cloud within every silver lining and makes sure to share her sad story with her friends. Sound familiar?

How can you balance the mix of reality versus positivity? By intentionally spending more time with people who exhibit a positive imagination. Perhaps it is the positive imagination that ultimately unleashes Einstein's higher level of thinking.

CHAPTER THREE
REVIEW QUESTIONS TO CONSIDER:

1. Name two reasons why Negative Nellie often commands your attention.
2. List three ways negative messages arrive on your doorstep.
3. What is the Hawthorne effect?
4. What can happen when you experience an amygdala hijack?

Chapter Four

The Man on the Moon Proves Einstein Correct

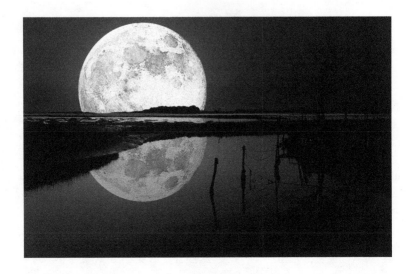

So far in this VAST Cognitive Replenishment primer we have discovered:

- In order to create the original solutions real life requires we need to replenish our minds with input that fuels our positive imagination.

- Both external and internal factors can assist or hinder us in achieving that goal.

- This VAST Cognitive Replenishment system supports us to be in right relationship to those essential factors.

We know that the same glass of chocolate milk can appear half-full or half-empty depending on our mood. What we often forget is that our perspective is dramatically influenced by the emotional content of what we ingest through our five senses. There is harmony and there is chaos in the world. There are peaceful and there are violent approaches to handling conflict. The impact of gratuitous messages or images of violence may be greater than you realize.

In 1996, Madeline Levine reviewed forty-years of prior research on the impact of media violence on children. What she found was that parents often "underestimate the impact of violent television on children and may be surprised at what children find upsetting" (Levine, 1996). She suggests that society is increasingly at risk not only for higher levels of violence, but for greater tolerance and acceptance of this violence.

And that was almost two decades ago...

The good news is that our neural gift of emotional connectivity works in both directions, making it just as easy to tune into the good vibes of the people around us. This creates a state of coherence. The HeartMath Institute defines coherence as "the harmonious flow of information, cooperation, and order among the subsystems of a larger system that allows for the emergence of more complex functions" (McCraty, 2003). Each of us experiences personal coherence on those days when we are in the flow of life and everything seems to be working smoothly.

Each of us can create a personal coherence strategy instead of ignoring the stressful impact of a continuously chaotic environment. Recognizing the dramatic areas and people in one's life is a powerful step toward effectively optimizing the quality of one's life.

Coherence is experienced when we feel peaceful after activities such as spending time in the gentle lap of nature, playing with a pet, or cuddling with a kindhearted companion. In those moments all of our systems work in harmony. Once we connect to this experience we can tip our inner scale in favor of coherence through simple, intentional replenishment techniques. For example, repeated exposure to positive people and messaging allows your brain to access the higher functions of the prefrontal cortex, which supports the development of your positive imagination and helps you solve the challenges you face in life (Goleman, 1995 & 2006).

"As far as being more effective, I find myself working less and making more. Maybe I am working more, but just have more fun so it seems like less." – L. M.

Positive imagination has fueled some of the finest achievements of individuals and humankind. Allow me to share one specific game-changing example.

In December of 1997, I attended an American Diabetes Association charity fundraiser in Houston honoring Chris Kraft Jr., NASA's first Flight Director for manned spaceflight during the Gemini Programs. That evening, Commander Eugene Cernan, the last man to walk on the moon, was going to introduce Mr. Kraft. I was eager to meet both men, for they embody my definition of a hero - people willing to risk their lives and pride to find solutions to complex problems meant to uplift humankind.

The room was packed with well-wishers. By chance, Mr. Kraft and Commander Cernan were posing for media photos at a space shuttle display close to our table. I seized the opportunity to ask them my burning question. I stood by patiently waiting to thank them for their bravery and as true gentlemen they were uncomfortable keeping a lady waiting. To my delight they stopped chatting with the press, acknowledged my presence and invited me over.

I then posed my question: in 1960, following President Kennedy's declaration that the USA would land a man on the moon and return him safely to the earth within the decade, had they understood at the time *how* that feat might be accomplished? The two gents smiled at one another. They then confided to me that at the onset no one at NASA had a clue. I too smiled at finally getting a credible answer, one that I had suspected all along.

In the early sixties, when President Kennedy declared that we would achieve this lofty goal we were forced to cooperate in order to solve problems that we did *not* yet know existed, in environments we had *never* experienced, under laws of physics that we *barely* understood. The odds of success were slim at best. Innovative problem solving was certainly required.

Hundreds, if not thousands, of people with diverse backgrounds, from varied disciplines, worked together to first imagine and then build the space program. They stretched the limits of human imagination. People just like you and I imagined into creation the thousands of solutions necessary for this goal to be accomplished. Brave men and women were willing to risk their lives to answer these bold questions and solve previously unimaginable challenges.

This dream required all the positive imagination we could muster. An uphill climb? Yes. But on July 20, 1969 they did it and as a result a new level of thinking was born.

Ever since that festive New Year's Eve, when I heard Mr. Kraft and Commander Cernan share their story, I have fully understood that to achieve our boldest successes as a species the unwavering positive imagination of a multitude of diverse people working together is required. This creates synergy. I believe that since we succeeded in reaching the moon and returning safely, we are capable of doing even greater things on this planet. But as Mr. Einstein stated, first we must advance our level of thinking. We can approach our challenges more easily after replenishing the cognitive functions that encourage and stimulate our positive imagination. Who knows what great achievements lay just beyond your current ability to imagine them? Mr. Einstein, Mr. Kraft and Commander Cernan are betting on us. They deserve a wholehearted response.

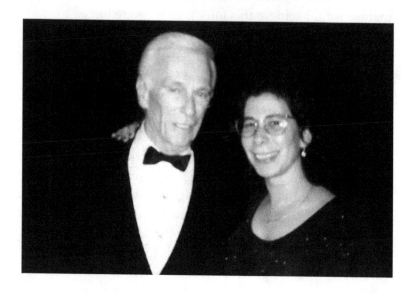

CHAPTER FOUR
REVIEW QUESTIONS TO CONSIDER:

1. What does cognitive replenishment fuel?
2. What feelings indicate an experience of personal coherence?
3. What has contributed to our boldest successes as a species?
4. How did the positive imagination of the NASA team enable us to reach to the moon?

CHAPTER FIVE

*The Subtle Yet Mysterious Workings of Your
Beautiful Brain*

Before we begin to discuss and practice The VAST Cognitive
Replenishment toolkit, this chapter will explain the impact
your daily choices have on your neural chemistry, which
significantly influences your quality of life.

There are some pertinent features of your beautiful
brain worth understanding. Our brain is constantly
releasing chemicals in reaction to stimuli. In proper balance
these neural chemicals, or hormones, keep the mind fit -
they can either hinder or enhance emotional health and
wellbeing. Below are some aspects of your mental world
that will make it easier to build your own unique Cognitive
Replenishment tool kit. Once you know a bit more about
these factors you can make the healthier choices that
ultimately work best for you.

DOSE
*Dopamine, Oxytocin, Serotonin and Endorphins are the fab four of
happy brain chemicals.*

In proper proportions this quartet aids your ability
to overcome negativity in your internal and external
environments. When DOSE is out of balance people often
feel overwhelmed, stressed, tired, depressed and/or
hopeless. Generally they have a bleak outlook on life. This
all stems from a brain depleted of the chemicals it needs to
thrive.

Individually:

Dopamine fuels the anticipation of happiness, as well as the desirability or addictive potential of activities through its secretion. Once released, dopamine serves several unique functions: it controls pleasure, is responsible for initiating seeking, wanting, desiring behaviors, motivation, arousal and goal-orientated behaviors, plus the feelings of satisfaction one has once an activity has been completed. On the flip side, dopamine is responsible for some activities turning into addictions. In a WebMD feature on the definition of addiction, psychiatrist Michael Brody, MD, set forth the following criteria:

The person needs more and more of a substance or behavior to keep them going.

If the person does not get more of the substance or behavior, they become irritable and miserable.

So it is our goal to understand this potential for addiction and create healthy, positive, balanced opportunities for dopamine to be released into our bodies.

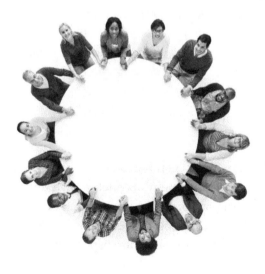

Oxytocin is known as the love, bond, tend and befriend hormone. It plays a key role in parental, sexual and partnership bonding behaviors. Elevated levels have even been found in owners bloodstreams after gazing into their canines' eyes (Nagasawa, 2009).

During research oxytocin has displayed some amazing effects on our daily social interactions, including the way it plays a role in our response to perceived danger.

In 2002, Klein and Taylor (two innovative women researchers at UCLA) suspected that,

> *"women have a larger behavioral repertoire than just fight or flight [...] it seems that when the hormone oxytocin is release as part of the stress responses in a woman, it buffers the fight or flight response and encourages her to tend children and gather with other women instead. When she actually engages in this tending or befriending, studies suggest that more oxytocin is released, which further counters stress and produces a calming effect. This calming response does not occur in men, [...] because testosterone---which men produce in high levels when they're under stress---seems to reduce the effects of oxytocin. Estrogen [...] seems to enhance it."*

(Berkowitz, 2002)

So it seems that when the hormone oxytocin interacts with estrogen it enhances the collaborative impulse in our species, leading not only to a greater chance of survival, but the ability to thrive. It is encouraging to know that under times of stress women are especially predisposed to problem solve cooperatively. In many cultures women gather the children and work together to overcome dangers and difficulties. The females of our species help to garner the cooperation of all concerned for the benefit of the community.

For those of you wondering what impact oxytocin has on the behavior of males it is this: the hormone promotes bonding and intimacy. Oxytocin is released during kissing, hugging, orgasm and other intimate moments between partners and serves to strengthen that bond. In one study, when men were given nasal doses of oxytocin, they rated the attractiveness of their partner as much higher compared to the attractiveness of other women with objectively similar characteristics (Hurlemann, 2013). Thus oxytocin in men appears to promote focus and bonding to a particular partner. Another way our biology works to ensure the survival of our species.

By working collaboratively to handle perceived threats we increase our chances of survival through what is referred to as divergent thinking. Divergent thinking is, "imaginative thinking, characterized by the generation of multiple possible solutions to a problem, often associated with creativity. The concept was introduced in 1946 by the US psychologist Joy Paul Guilford"(Oxford Reference Dictionary). Synergistic acts are facilitated in part by oxytocin, as demonstrated by the way the females of our species cooperatively respond to stress. Fascinating and exciting to think that Taylor and Klein's research on oxytocin shows that cooperation has been an adaptive strategy for our species. Despite any sexist stereotypes, cooperation is just one part (a very important part indeed) of the feminine contribution to problem solving.

Please do not mistake cooperation as a sign that you are

not strong enough to handle situations on your own. The truth is the strategy of collaboration embodies strength not weakness.

Serotonin is a neurotransmitter that affects your mood, social behavior, sleep pattern, memory, sexual desire and sexual functioning. It also plays a vital role in regulating anxiety and happiness. Some recreational drugs and antidepressants elevate serotonin levels. This often results in a decreased libido.

Serotonin has an important connection to stress and anxiety. Having healthy amounts of serotonin makes you better able to cope with stress and not feel anxious. However, stress and anxiety can deplete our stores of serotonin leaving us even more vulnerable to cognitive depletion. Thus, boosting your serotonin levels is an important step in your Cognitive Replenishment. In chapter seven, we will discuss some ways you can start replenishing your mind through implementing "mind moves".

Endorphins are the feel-good proteins produced by your brain, designed to relieve stress and enhance pleasure. They lead to feelings of euphoria and they decrease the perception of pain. High endorphin levels help you cope with sustained physical activity and exhaustion. Endorphins are the body's naturally occurring painkiller. All creatures, including single-celled organisms, produce endorphins. Endorphins help you cope with stress and aid your Cognitive Replenishment practice.

A variety of things have been shown to release endorphins including: exercise, sex, ginseng, dark chocolate and even scents, such as lavender or vanilla. In 1991, in order to address the anxiety often experienced by cancer patients during their MRI scans, Dr. William H. Redd of Sloan-Kettering Cancer Center tested the effects of five fragrances on eighty-five patients undergoing the procedure. Heliotropin, a vanilla-like aroma was rated the most relaxing. The patients exposed to heliotropin reported a sixty-three-percent reduction in anxiety and claustrophobia, compared to those not exposed to any fragrance. This study prompted Sloan-Kettering to include vanilla fragrances as a standard part of MRI scans. (Redd, 1991)

In proper balance DOSE provides the chemical catalysts to fuel your overall sense of confidence and well-being.

The Mirror Neuron
Where emotional connection begins

In 1992, while studying Macaque monkeys' brain activity, Italian researchers discovered something remarkable. During the researcher's gelato break, the monkey's premotor cortex activity was identical to what it would be if it were reaching for the gelato itself. How could that be, as the monkeys were merely observing the researchers eat the gelato? It led to the discovery of what we call mirror neurons. This special class of brain cell fires not only when an individual performs an action, but when the individual observes the action as well. In Daniel Goleman's book, *Social Intelligence*, he explains,

> *"Since the first sighting of mirror neurons in monkeys, the same systems have been discovered in the human brain… when a laser thin electrode monitored a single neuron in an awake person, the neuron fired both when the person anticipated*

> *pain- a pinprick- and when merely seeing someone*
> *else receive a pinprick- a neural snapshot of*
> *empathy in action."* (Goleman, 2007, pg. 41)

So we can literally feel each other's pain and joy.

Daniel Stern, an American Psychiatrist specializing in mother-infant relations, adds that mirror neurons are present to ensure those around you will experience the feelings you convey. Emotional connections exist on conscious and subconscious levels. So, what happens when those around are incessantly sad, or terrified, or the last four movies you saw on Netflix were horror films? This may be a good time for you to refresh that menu to include some comedies and kid-fun movies. In this day and age of instant information, we must each consider if a regular entertainment and news diet of fear, shame, horror, darkness and sadness has unintended consequences on our emotional, physical or spiritual health. For you to decide and to know.

The more you decide to focus your attention on the good stuff around you, the easier it becomes: the food on the table, children's laughter, puppy antics, a warm shower, a clean glass of water with a simple yet delicious dinner, coming in second at the bowling league (and feeling inspired to do even better next time), school plays, berries in the backyard, bluebirds and squirrels visiting, neighbors sharing their bumper crop of squash, volunteering to help those in need... These are just a few examples of the loving kindness you experience throughout the day *if* you to choose to notice it. As you recognize the good stuff that is already present in your life you will be amazed at how often new good starts appearing. Same life, different point of view.

The Amygdala Hijack
When our primitive instincts prevail

In his 1995 groundbreaking book on emotional intelligence, Daniel Goleman explains how anger can get out of hand, or hijacked. The amygdala is the part of the limbic system, responsible for passion, emotional behavior and motivation. Among other things, it stores your intense emotionally-laden memories. According to Goleman, "The amygdala's extensive web of neural connections allows it, during an emotional emergency, to capture and drive much of the rest of the brain- including the rational mind" (Goleman, 1995, pg. 17).

An amygdala hijack happens when your response to a perceived threat is immediate, overwhelming and out of proportion to the problem. This happens because the brain has been triggered to respond to what it mistakenly believes is a significant hazard. This amygdala hijack feels like a runaway stagecoach barreling down the road towards trouble, causing you to lose control. The experience of emotional flooding "is a self-perpetuated emotional hijack" that can fuel rage, violence and even panic (Goleman, 1995, pg. 139). Such an angry person might benefit from a squirt of oxytocin, the "tend and befriend" neural-chemical elixir.

The amygdala hijack impacts your world as you overreact to a person or problem with a survival-specific strategy such as anger, violence, panic, shame or blame. During the perceived threat of danger your rational prefrontal cortex is banished. During an amygdala hijack your brain decides that self-control is less valuable than emotional intensity or the immediate gratification of a violent reaction. Ever witness yourself or someone else crossing the line during an angry outburst?

When I was fourteen-years-old a supposed friend lied about me to my closest friends and family. In doing so, he temporarily damaged my relationship with my parents, my sister and my boyfriend. I was livid at his deceit and deception. It took three adult lifeguards to hold me down and prevent me from hurting that boy. I became blind with rage. That's an amygdala hijack. We make fools of ourselves during an amygdala hijack due to our brain's inability to access our higher reasoning skills.

Goleman proceeds to point out that "anger builds on anger" (Goleman, 1995, pg. 61). Anger is a response to a perceived endangerment of our physical or emotional selves. Real or imagined, such threats can trigger an emotional flooding. Dolf Zillman, of the University of Alabama, confirmed what we each have witnessed, anger builds upon itself. Zillman sees escalating anger as "a sequence of provocations each triggering an excitatory response that dissipates slowly. In this sequence every successive anger-provoking thought or perception becomes a mini trigger for amygdala-driven surges of catecholamine, each building on the hormonal momentum of those that went before"(Zillman, 1979). Goleman adds, when "anger builds upon anger: the emotional brain heats up. By then rage, unhampered by reason, easily erupts into violence"(Goleman, 1995, pg. 61).

If we do not "cool down" our subsequent outbursts gain further intensity, often erupting into violent behaviors. This is why it is referred to as a crime of passion.

By practicing a few of the Cognitive Replenishment techniques suggested in this course you will learn to recognize these moments and more easily return control to the rational, problem-solving prefrontal cortex. That portion of your brain acts as the executive branch, for it differentiates conflicting thoughts, allows you to work toward a defined goal, identifies the future consequences of present actions and suppresses the impulse to seek immediate gratification. In short, the prefrontal cortex civilizes us with the gift of cooperation, rational thought and self-control. These higher problem solving functions are the gifts we need to reclaim after an amygdala hijack.

Memes
Ideas that catch like wildfire

The Oxford English Dictionary defines a meme as:

> *"An element of a culture or system of behavior that may be considered to be passed from one individual to another by nongenetic means, especially imitation."*

Wikipedia adds:

> *"A meme acts as a unit for carrying cultural ideas, symbols, or practices that can be transmitted from one mind to another through writing, speech, gestures, rituals, or other imitable phenomena with a mimicked theme. Supporters of the concept regard memes as cultural analogues to genes in that they self-replicate, mutate, and respond to selective pressures."*

What memes are you perpetuating? An idea can take root and spread like wildfire throughout the human brain trust. Something that trends on Twitter is an example of a meme catching fire. Of course memes have unintended consequences, for as Dr. David Hawkins points out in *Power versus Force,* there is no way for the human brain to discern truth from untruth (Hawkins, 1995, pg. 35).

Once an idea, true or false, healthy or unhealthy, is unleashed, it can catch the collective imagination and spread, creating either coherence or disruption in its wake. We have all heard of Chicken Little who mistakenly creates hysteria among her friends by stating that the sky is falling. In truth, it was only an acorn. Another example is the erroneous belief that eating carrots can help you see in the dark. This meme actually comes from intentionally disseminated WWII propaganda. The British developed a new radar detection system and in order to hide this game-changing technology from the Germans they spread the myth that British pilots had exceptional night-vision due to eating so many carrots. The carrots had nothing to do with the British pilot's success, but the meme persists to this day (Smith, 2013).

Of course a meme is only as powerful as its ability to command your attention. It is a wise person who knows where, when and what to pay attention to.

Embracing every message that is presented to us does not always serve to inform, uplift or resolve anything.

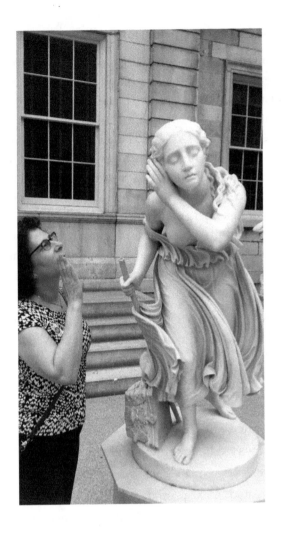

"So much of our perception
is conditioned by our fears and our desires.
We must learn to see things
That others cannot see.
Then we must assure them of the beauty hidden there."
— *The Sage's Tao Te Ching, (Page 55).*

Chronic stress and your cortisol levels

Cortisol, a steroid hormone that is produced within your adrenal glands, regulates blood pressure, glucose metabolism, insulin release, immune function and inflammatory response. It also balances the body's electrolyte chemistry. Cortisol is meant to improve your chance of survival when a threat, real or imagined, is perceived. Even small increases in cortisol levels have a positive impact on survival when you are facing difficulties, by causing quick energy, enhanced memory function, increased immunity and desensitization to pain. Once the threat is assessed and handled, cortisol levels are meant to decrease, as the body experiences a relaxation response that returns it to its normal state.

However, when cortisol levels in the bloodstream stay elevated for prolonged periods of time, negative effects occur such as:

- Impaired cognitive performance
- Suppressed thyroid function
- Elevated blood sugar levels
- Decreased bone mineral density
- Decrease in muscle mass
- Elevated blood pressure
- Lowered immunity and inflammatory responses in the body, causing delayed wound healing, and other negative health consequences

An increase in fat deposits in abdominal organs, which is associated with a greater risk of health problems. Some of the health risks are: heart attacks, strokes, the development of metabolic syndrome, higher levels of "bad" cholesterol (LDL) and lower levels of "good" cholesterol (HDL) (Mayo Clinic, 2013).

To keep cortisol levels healthy and under control, the body needs to return to its relaxed state after a fight-or-flight response occurs. But that does not happen if your attention is continually commandeered by the negative messages from news feeds, TV and radio ads, workplace downsizing memos, violent video games, incessant TV murder mysteries, your Negative Nellie neighbor or a horror movie advertisement. If you are always agitated about the state of your world and rarely experience a relaxation response, it sets you up for the health risks listed above, which are associated with a state of chronic stress.

A 2014 article on women and stress from the American Psychological Society, discovered that "in the past month, more women than men reported signs and symptoms of stress. Significantly more women experienced a lack of interest, motivation or energy, feelings of being overwhelmed and the inability to control the important things in their lives" (American Psychological Society, 2014, pg.3).

Despite the challenges they report, women appear to be more aware than men of the impact stress can have on their lives. Women are more likely to say stress has a strong or very strong impact on their physical and mental health. They are also more likely than men to say that a psychologist can help with stress management.

Although women acknowledge the problem more often, we all need to learn to relax our bodies using stress management techniques. We need to incorporate lifestyle changes designed to keep us balanced and able to react intelligently to the common stressors of modern life.

In conclusion, we humans are wired to experience each other's emotional state, be it coherence or dissonance.

Feelings of joy, peace and love create coherence. In contrast, being bombarded with shame, fear and violence can create a dissonance in our bodies, hijacking our ability to solve problems in non-violent ways, bypassing our higher reasoning. If we stay in that state of dissonance for too long chronic stress will begin to compromise our health.

What can you do to minimize the disruption of joy experienced in your inner and outer worlds? How can you intentionally stimulate the fab four happy brain chemicals in order to minimize the impact of incessant chaos and outrage? One step towards Cognitive Replenishment is to identify the factors that unwittingly create cognitive depletion within your mental realm.

Our next chapter will help you do just that.

CHAPTER FIVE
REVIEW QUESTIONS TO CONSIDER:

1. Name the fab four of happy brain chemicals (aka DOSE)?

2. What is the connection between mirror neurons and emotional contagion?

3. What occurs when oxytocin interacts with estrogen?

4. What is a meme?

5. Name two outcomes of chronic stress.

Chapter Six

Cognitive Exhaustion – The New Norm?

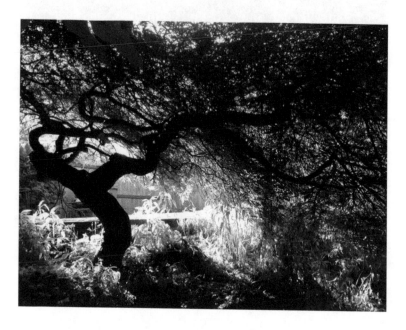

Serving as a success coach over the past thirty-years has shown me that many clients experience mental exhaustion even after they get plenty of sleep, eat relatively well and experience joy in their lives. On the very first page of this program we stated the VAST Institute wholeheartedly believes that the way to significantly enhance your sense of well-being and quality of life is to:

1. Nourish your mind

2. Develop a positive imagination

3. Take command of where you place your attention

4. Set healthier boundaries.

When you practice and paint these four skills into your daily landscape the cognitive fatigue begins to lift. Before people can imagine and generate a life that promotes their physical, professional and emotional well-being they need to identify what can often be the invisible factors that contribute to their cognitive weariness.

At VAST we refer to these as cognitive depletors.

Here are some of the most common and recurring cognitive depletors. All of these depletors were discovered, because they were patterns I saw again and again while working with hundreds of VAST clients over the years. Although this list is not complete, it is meant to get you thinking about where cognitive depletion shows up in your world. Identifying these issues is a bold and powerful first step in making more replenishing choices.

"Michelle's approach to coaching has served me well. Hers is a 'whole life' view and approach... I was sometimes impatient with some of the conversations we had that touched on topics such as my unwillingness to take care of myself, my ways of interacting in key relationships in my life, or the choices I had made so far in life. Instead, I wanted to talk about how to get my marketing plan underway! Fortunately, Michelle knew where we needed to go first. I was patient with the process and with myself. My work with Michelle has resulted in a near seamless integration of my personal and professional lives as well as my internal and external selves." —E.S.

Cognitive Depletors

Overstimulation

Overstimulation is especially challenging for the part of the population that Elaine Aron, PhD, calls the highly sensitive person (HSP). Commonly referred to as shy, the HSP needs plenty of alone time to recharge. "We're all social beings who enjoy and must depend on others. But many HSPs avoid people who come in the overstimulating packages – the strangers, the big parties, the crowds. For most HSPs this is a smart strategy. In a highly stimulating, demanding world, everyone has to establish priorities" (Aron, 1996, pg. 97). After staring at a computer screen for hours, reading a multitude of Facebook posts, watching a variety of news feeds, wondering if your department will be re-orged, or watching dystopian entertainment, even the toughest among us can feel depleted. Overstimulation can also be the result of a lack of mental rest, quietude or exposure to nature.

24/7 connectivity

There is a new addict in town and he is connected 24/7. This person never eats or sits without a device in front of him and interrupts contact with people to respond to the relentless flood of emails, texts, Facebook posts and voicemail. While another person is terrified that if she is not checking her devices 24/7 she will miss something essential and pay dearly for it. Fear underpins these behaviors. Such hypervigilance and fear leaves no time for rest and recovery. As a result, rehab clinics for device addiction have emerged to support those who struggle to establish boundaries regarding technology. New boundaries are required to navigate new cultural norms. We discuss these types of questions as well as places to find solutions in chapter seven.

Inability to set cognitive limits or boundaries

Although it is an important skill to decline situations that are harmful to us, it is not always realistic or possible.

Sometimes you just can't say no to a boss, or cannot ignore the realities of a difficult economy. Some circumstances are beyond our control. Managing these difficulties and depletors while keeping track of things that are constantly changing can be exhausting. Sometimes the people who are supposed to lead us prove inept and that in and of itself is depleting. It is especially important in these instances to develop a Cognitive Replenishment practice. Learn how to set healthy limits and advocate for yourself. If this is new to you we suggest starting with the book *Boundaries,* by Anne Katherine, a great primer on this type of self-care.

FUD = (Fear, Uncertainty and Doubt)

This negative messaging would erode even Mickey Mouses' confidence. FUD appears in the guise of put-downs, sarcasm, blame, victimization or outrage. It is often presented as a joke to keep you off balance, tense and ill at ease. People who perpetuate FUD are often seen as bullies or narcissists, who use this technique to establish their superiority and control over those around them.

- **Confusion** – mixed messages, hypocrisy.
  This occurs when the people around you say one thing and do another. At work, when the mission statement of the company speaks of fairness and respect, but people around you are yelled at, embarrassed and ignored, it causes confusion. When the company motto stresses customer care, but employees are not given the authority to help their customers, it sends a mixed message. According to VAST, integrity is consistency in thought, word and deed. People who have integrity can be counted on to do what they say and say what they will do. Honest, simple and highly effective.

- **Emotional distress**

    When at home or work you are asked to participate in one dramatic crisis after another, but the cause of this chaos is never addressed by those who profess to want to improve things. When folks like this are around, you have to continually overcome the drama, give them reassurance and prove you like, care or love them. These are the relationships in our lives that demand an inordinate amount of our energy. Without healthy boundaries their drama and crisis can be a source of ongoing emotional distress.

- **Disrespectful treatment at home or work.**

    When those in positions of authority abuse the trust of the workers, family members, or citizens who count on them. When certain groups of people are treated better than others based on their job title or superficial characteristics. The Workplace Bullying Institute reported in their 2014 survey that twenty-seven-percent of their respondents have directly experienced current or past abusive conduct at work. While seventy-two-percent of the American public are aware of workplace bullying, seventy-two-percent of employers deny, discount, encourage, rationalize or defend it (Namie, 2014). A study conducted in Italy found that workers exposed to workplace bullying had a higher sickness absenteeism rate as compared to non-exposed workers (Campanini, 2013).

- **Negativity around you** in the guise of people, words used and ideas circulated.

    Does their worldview replenish or deplete you energetically? Do they see all as hopeless, painful, and inevitably destructive? No matter what solutions you propose they are immediately dismissed as impossible. This type of person succeeds in stimulating your negative imagination, because it comforts them to be cynical.

Ironically, I have found (and many of my clients have confirmed) that "the same associates who were most opposed at the onset are now the biggest supporters" of this process (A.L.). Often it is the most negative among us who derive the greatest benefit and undergo a dramatic transformation from a Cognitive Replenishment practice.

Exposure to recurring messages and images of gore, hurt, harm, hopelessness and violence.

Web MD advisor Elizabeth Heuback cautions parents of 0-3-year-olds that young children lack a context for the violence shown and do not understand it. Yet, it still frightens them. "Ideally say the experts, it is best to avoid exposing very young children to violent images altogether" (Heuback, 2007). Perhaps their nervous system requires some insulation from negative, emotional memes. As we grow and mature our ability to process the violence shown to us increases, yet we still need to focus on getting our brain chemistry balanced. A cognitively depleted adult's ability to process these negative messages and/or images though, is going to be compromised. It is wise to reduce our exposure to messages and images of violence, hopelessness or despair, because you will unintentionally absorb their downbeat vibe. This is one of the ways that emotional contagion works.

Cognitive depletion leads to a state of sustained stress

and lack of rest for your mind. Always having a screen in front of us compromises our ability to reset our brain chemistry. We must each learn to allow the relaxation response to kick in after handling a perceived threat. If you do not allow your mind and body to rest and refresh you wear it down. Therefore this is the age where we need to develop new types of cognitive boundaries.

Boundaries are about setting limits. Limits on how much hurt, harm and unnecessary suffering our individual nervous system can process in the name of entertainment. Limits on the negativity we unintentionally soak up in the course of a given day from colleagues, friends, family members and clever corporations marketing to our insecurities. It is an opportunity to advocate for what is in our best interest. In my experience the world reflects back to me what I imagine and where I pay my attention. Let us use healthy boundaries to create more harmonious options and outcomes.

"Building boundaries can work from outside in or inside out. You can build boundaries with conscious effort and this will change you on the inside — or, you can change your insides and the boundaries will automatically form. You can set deliberate limits to protect what you care about — or, they will spring up by themselves when you focus your whole self on what matters to you most" (Katherine, 2013, pg. 13).

Sometimes boundary issues can be very subtle and insidious. Boundary violations are often the result of habitual responses learned over many years, leading us to choices that are not in our best interest, but that we feel we must make to ensure our success or well-being. We don't always see that we have options, but there usually are.

"My career tendency had always been to say 'yes' to what was offered to me. The consulting environment in which I had worked for twenty-years was one of scarcity... Through Michelle's coaching I developed a confident, self-respectful, proactive business approach... I developed different messages about myself...and my boundaries in terms of what I want and what I will accept." – V.M.

Let us now turn our attention to creating healthier cognitive boundaries by exploring how to craft a personal Cognitive Replenishment practice.

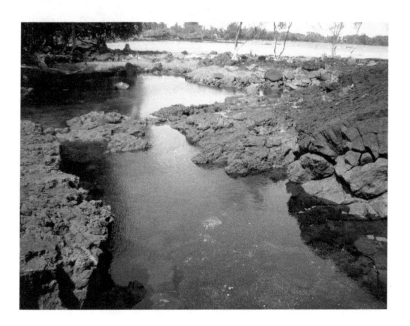

CHAPTER SIX
REVIEW QUESTIONS TO CONSIDER:

1. What does FUD stand for?

2. Name three ways to enhance your sense of wellbeing.

3. Name two cognitive depletors that you have experienced.

4. Why is it important to set cognitive boundaries?

NOTES AND INSIGHTS

CHAPTER SEVEN

The Care and Feeding of Your Healthy Mind is a Laughing Matter

This chapter will share a total of eighteen options from which you can choose to build your own Cognitive Replenishment practice.

I have discovered that intentionally building my positive imagination via a Cognitive Replenishment practice can bear magical fruit. One example that comes to mind was when I was pregnant with my daughter. She was my first child and I wanted to birth her without the use of drugs. While I researched my options, it didn't take me long to discover that this choice would require all the positive imagination I could muster. Most people thought I was crazy, or said it couldn't be done. The lessons of this situation can be applied to all feats large and small that others' say is impossible for you. Don't believe them.

I had a lot to overcome. First, there was the negative self-talk that moving a watermelon-sized object through my birth canal was impossible and I would explode. Then there were the horror stories of well-meaning friends, who had experienced difficult births. They often said to me with sincerity that a natural, drug-free childbirth was a combination of insane and impossible. This was when my Cognitive Replenishment practice as outlined in this chapter served me well.

I decided to trust my instincts and give my baby the gift of what others thought impossible. Babies have been born drug-free for thousands of years and most of the time it worked out. I affirmed constantly that I could trust my healthy body. If I had needed to make other arrangements I most certainly would have. But I was determined to give this my best shot. I wanted to be awake to welcome my daughter into the world, so I read up on research that supported drug-free methods (McCutcheon- Rosegg, Ingraham, 1984). I avoided all the Negative Nellies and sought inspiration from those who had successfully done what I dreamed to do. This allowed me to imagine a terrific outcome.

When the day arrived, I had a birth plan that my doctor had previously approved, detailing my preferences. The bed was surrounded by those rooting for our success, and when my daughter emerged both she and I were victorious, awake and fully connected.

We did what others thought impossible. Impossible for them, but mine to imagine, claim and create. This is the power of a Cognitive Replenishment practice.

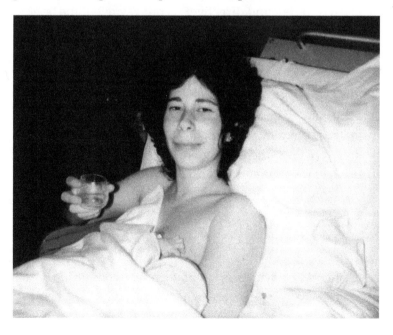

Let me share some of the ways to build your very own.

About two decades ago I first heard of a man named Norman Cousins who wrote the classic, *Anatomy of an Illness as Perceived by the Patient.* What caught my attention was how Mr. Cousins, who was suffering from a serious, crippling illness, employed laughter as a tool to heal himself. Wow! I love the thought that giggling can be a potent self-healing force - the type of tool to support the care and feeding of a healthy mind.

Based on our earlier neural chemical discussion, perhaps Cousins was intentionally boosting his dose of DOSE with laughter. Or perhaps he was spending time imagining a dance with the kindhearted and wonderful nurse. Or, perhaps he was meditating and allowing his thoughts to focus on awe, gratitude and joy, which are emotions associated with personal coherence. Perhaps he chose to surround himself with mostly those who sincerely saw and supported his healing directive. As one review of the book stated, Mr. Cousins forged,

"An unusual collaboration with his physician, and together they were able to beat the odds. The doctor's genius was in helping his patient to use his own powers: laughter, courage, and tenacity. The patient's talent was in mobilizing his body's own natural resources, proving what an effective healing tool the mind can be. This remarkable story of the triumph of the human spirit is truly inspirational reading." (Amazon.com review of *Anatomy of an Illness as Perceived by the Patient*)

The whole affair seemed miraculous when the book was written two-decades ago. Mr. Cousins' unscientific results fostered a scientific interest by the medical community, inspiring whole-person care, which evolved into the fields of integrative and lifestyle medicine. The neural science is catching up to our intuitive wisdom that laughter is good for the soul. Now we are able to see detailed brain activity through images produced by CT or MRI scans.

So what other helpful activities could replenish your brain chemistry, reduce your stress and stimulate that positive imagination? Over the years we have seen great benefit from the following. Find the ones that appeal to you. You may identify and add some of your own.

VAST COGNITIVE REPLENISHMENT "MIND MOVES" *for you to play with*

Laughter

Norm Cousins' wisdom led to the scientific investigation of the impact of "mirthful laughter" on our physiology (Berk, 1989). In the 1980s, Dr. Lee Berk found that even the anticipation of a humorous movie can significantly increase both beta-endorphins and human growth hormone (HGH), which support immunity.

If laughter can help us heal on a physical, emotional and spiritual level, then can ongoing exposure to angst and depravity harm us? The UCLA Facebook study, which manipulated the happy or sad messages sent to their users, supports that premise. If you manipulate people's emotional state you ultimately affect their choices.

To combat being unintentionally dragged into someone else's emotional landscape, it is best to understand the skills that comprise emotional intelligence.

Emotional Intelligence

Emotional intelligence, simply put, is the ability to understand emotional states and be able to work effectively with them. Emotional intelligence can act as a social lubricant and make the experience of interacting with other people go more smoothly.

Emotionally intelligent folk:

1. Know their emotions
2. Manage their emotions
3. Motivate themselves
4. Recognize emotions in others
5. Handle their relationships in a socially competent manner. (Goleman, 1997, pg. 43-44)

Integrating the skills listed above leads to a state of personal responsibility, appreciation and coherence. That in turn boosts our fab four, DOSE. Lovely how that works.

Brain Nutrition

What you put into your body fuels your brain and mind, so the content and quality of it matters a great deal. A nutritious diet full of good proteins, fats and complex carbohydrates, will support healthy cognitive function. You can learn more about this from the Harvard School of Public Health's nutrition blog: www.hsph.harvard.edu/nutritionsource.

Safe Physical Touch

It is a wonderful thing to feel safe to cuddle with another dear, sweet human being. Experiencing a caring, comforting and non-threatening interaction with another person is beneficial.

Physical touch is necessary for infants and children for normal growth and development. According to Harlow's research, a lack of physical touch can lead to severe emotional disturbances, triggering a "failure to thrive" reaction in baby monkeys (Harlow, 1958). During his studies on the developmental impact of physical touch on rhesus monkeys, he discovered that cuddling provided infants with the reassurance and security needed to keep normal development on track. A failure to thrive syndrome is also reported in children who have had a loss of physical touch or emotional bonding with their caregiver. Symptoms in children include: diminished physical growth and a delay in achieving basic mental, social motor skills (Barbero, 1967, Bauchner, 2007).

So create clear boundaries with a safe "hug buddy" to get that need met in a comfortable and loving manner. Incorporate more affection into your relationships, romantic or platonic.

Smiling

> "If you smile at me I will understand, 'cause
> that is something everybody, everywhere
> does in the same language."
> —Crosby, Stills & Nash

The simple act of smiling benefits both your brain chemistry and social capital. It elevates the feel good chemicals in your brain as it signals a desire to connect with others in a positive way. A heartfelt smile is a highly effective short cut to world peace. It is a sincere, cost effective way to put people at ease and open your heart to total strangers. Smiling lovingly at other people's children, especially those unlike you, can be particularly effective.

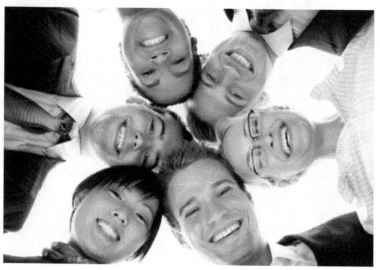

The world is warmed one kindhearted smile at a time. Even a "Negative Nellie" can experience some amazing benefits from a forced smile. A smile created mechanically by placing chopsticks in a subject's mouth still brightened up their brain chemistry. And, it has been discovered that a Duchenne smile, one where lips and the corners of the eyes twinkle, stimulates the brain to produce neural chemicals that foster a happier mood (Ekman, 1990).

"Findings revealed that all smiling participants, regardless of whether they were aware of smiling, had lower heart rates during stress recovery than the neutral group

did, with a slight advantage for those with Duchenne smiles." (Kraft, 2012)

Taken all together with our earlier discussion on emotional contagion, as well as studies by Marco Iacoboni of UCLA that show our brains are wired for sociability, it becomes clear that something as simple as a smile can have a huge impact. In particular, if someone observes another person smiling, mirror neurons in their brain will light up as if they were the one smiling (Iacoboni, 2008). Perhaps this is nature's way of positively stimulating even grumpy people's brain chemistry.

So go ahead and smile, especially in those moments when you may not feel like it. After a bit of time not only will your own mood lighten, but you will simultaneously trigger positive feelings in the people around you.

> "Peace begins with a smile. Smile five times
> a day at someone you don't really want to
> smile at all. Do it for peace."
> — Mother Teresa

Friendships

> "Friends are the people you pick to be your
> cheerleaders, fans and buddies. They root for
> your success. They are kind, generous and
> appreciate your unique qualities. They share
> their cookies. They really like you!" — M.S.

Friendships, like all relationships, can range from healthy to toxic.

Earlier we discussed how positive and negative messages elicit either a positive or negative physiological response, which can ultimately impact our health. This concept also applies to the friends who are creating these messages.

One study showed that friends who talk excessively about problems can actually increase one another's stress levels - a well-known contributor to heart disease (Reblin, 2008). Research has found that inflammation is another primary contributor to heart disease, as elevated levels of inflammation are evident in the bodies of those with heart disease (Black, 2002). However, research has also found that people who enjoy close support from friends and family display reduced levels of these same inflammatory markers (Cadzow, 2009). So go hug a friend, it's good for your heart.

Dr. Jan Yaeger Ph.D. has identified trust, empathy, honesty, confidentiality, acceptance, and appropriate boundaries as the six essential elements of healthy friendship. If there are ongoing problems in any of these areas, a toxic or dysfunctional relationship may result. When things are difficult, friends help smooth out the rough patches and can talk you off an emotional ledge. Men and women studied during a particularly difficult time in their life demonstrated a reduction in their pulse and blood pressures when they had a supportive friend by their side. As a matter of fact, friendships can even encourage healthier lifestyle choices. It was shown to be easier for people to eat fruits and vegetable, exercise regularly and quit smoking, if they had a network of friends and family members on their side (Current Opinion in Psychiatry, 2008).

A three-year study conducted in Sweden of more than thirteen-thousand men and women found that those who had few or no close friends had a fifty-percent increase in their risk of having a heart attack. Women who participated in a two-year study by the same researchers, who reported the lowest levels of emotional support, were twice as likely to die during the study (Eng, 2001).

Friends are the family you choose. Choose wisely. Surround yourself with people who are happy for your success as well as their own. Spend as much time with healthy, positive, kind people as you can. Friends who have a positive outlook, are respectful and appreciate others can add years to your life.

Whether for a minute or a month, that type of replenishing interaction with another person enhances personal coherence and self-esteem. You are able to relax around them, because they have your best interest at heart. And, while you are at it, make sure you treat others with the same level of respect and kindness you would like to receive.

We at the VAST Institute define a healthy adult relationship as one within which each person is able to learn, grow and thrive as their unique, whole and best self. The information in this workbook can support you in building healthier relationships. As you can see, friendships possess both great health benefits and perhaps a few good laughs. For as Kahil Gibran said, "Friendship is always a sweet responsibility, never an opportunity".

For those interested in building some additional relationship muscles check out our VAST Healthy Adult Relationships online programs and teleconferences at www.vastinstitute.com

Music

Almost everyone enjoys music. Not only is it pleasurable, it has been shown to have a positive effect on our brains and health as well. Listening to music that you like has been associated with sleeping better, alleviating chronic pain from conditions like arthritis, decreasing stress and helping to manage anxiety and depression (Allred et al, 2010; de Niet et al, 2009; Lin et al, 2011). The way music affects our brains is by stimulating the production of dopamine while simultaneously bolstering our immune systems.

Music also taps into a universal human experience that can inspire cooperation. It was shown in one study that,

"Among participants, the researchers found synchronization in several key brain areas, and similar brain activity patterns in different people who listen to the same music. This suggests that the participants not only perceive the music the same way, but, despite whatever personal differences they brought to the table, there's a level on which they share a common experience...The results also reflect the power of music to unite people." (Landau, 2013)

Many of us have the experience of finding that the songs we loved during our adolescences are prized throughout our lives. In that instance music may help bring an entire generation of people together through a shared message. These messages can be positive or negative, you decided. Whatever music does to stimulate, calm and inspire you, allow music to be a cost effective way to soothe a rough day.

I often spend time working with birdsong music playing in the background. It relaxes and soothes my mind, heart and soul to hear the joyful chatter of birds in the woods.

Take a Vacation from Social Media

Electronic devices like smartphones and all manner of social media platforms have been shown to trigger addictive behaviors and psychological dependencies in vulnerable individuals. The effects can look a lot like a gambling addiction (Rauh, 2011). But even for those who don't get hooked on compulsively checking emails or status updates, staying constantly online can make anyone feel anxious, depressed, overwhelmed and cognitively depleted.

> "Peter Whybrow, the director of the Semel Institute for Neuroscience and Human Behavior at UCLA, argues that 'the computer is like electronic cocaine,' fueling cycles of

mania followed by depressive stretches. The Internet 'leads to behavior that people are conscious is not in their best interest and does leave them anxious and does make them act compulsively,' says Nicholas Carr, whose book *The Shallows*, about the Web's effect on cognition, was nominated for a Pulitzer Prize. It 'fosters our obsessions, dependence, and stress reactions,' adds Larry Rosen, a California psychologist who has researched the Net's effect for decades." (Dokoupil, 2012)

The internet and social media are tools, thus they are not inherently good or bad for us. It all comes down to how we use (or abuse) them in our daily lives. Most importantly, the boundaries we have with social media matter, or without them we won't feel in control of the compulsion to stay connected 24/7 (Katherine, 2013).

For the benefit of your own Cognitive Replenishment, VAST suggests you take a break from social media every once in a while, even for just a day. Work to create healthy boundaries with social media in your personal and professional life. Get comfortable saying "no" or turning off your devices. Gain back your control by making conscious choices instead of giving into compulsive pressures. There are many people taking vacations from social media who have shared their advice and resources, such as Justin Hempel from Wired magazine.

If you are still unsure if staring at a computer screen for endless hours is bad for you, perhaps the findings from a 2011 *Journal of the American College of Cardiology* will change your perception. Their research found that time spent in front of a TV or computer screen was associated with a higher risk of death, independent of the subject's physical activity level. Additional studies associate TV and computer screen time with loss of empathy and lack of altruism (Weinstein, 2009).

If you would like some help imagining what taking a break from social media might look like for you we highly recommend Anne Katherine's book *Boundaries in an Overconnected World*.

Set Healthier Boundaries

> "Good fences make good neighbors."
> – Robert Frost

Healthy boundaries are about setting limits with people in a way that protects us and enhances our wellbeing. When we neglect to create boundaries, negativity in all its forms can impact the quality of our lives. As we discussed in chapter three, the world is often presented in a very intense and negative light by the media, ad campaigns, horror movies and ongoing wars. This negativity can take the form of media sensationalism, graphic violence or chaotic family members who endlessly focus on problems rather than solutions. During an interview in 2008 with Scientific American, emotional contagion researcher Marco Iacoboni was asked about the impact violent movies, television programs and video games have on us. He said,

> "I believe we should be more careful about what we watch. This is a tricky argument, of course, because it forces us to reconsider our long cherished ideas about free will, and may potentially have repercussions on free speech. There is convincing behavioral evidence linking media violence with

imitative violence. Mirror neurons provide
a plausible neurobiological mechanism
that explains why being exposed to media
violence leads to imitative violence. What
should we do about it? Although it is
obviously hard to have a clear and definitive
answer, it is important to openly discuss
this issue and hopefully reach some kind of
'societal agreement' on how to limit media
violence without limiting free speech."

It is important to be aware of the unintended neural-
chemical consequences of prolonged exposure to violent
images and begin to establish personal, physical, emotional
and cognitive boundaries. This may look like watching
a light-hearted movie instead of one with gratuitous
violence. I recently went to see an action movie that was
so graphically violent, I became physically ill and even my
husband, who loves action movies, felt squeamish. You can
choose to read historical fiction instead of watching hours
of TV punctuated by pharmaceutical commercials every
five-minutes. You can sit in your backyard or walk the dog.
Take a mental vacation (braincation) or spend time with an
inspiring friend, music or book. This will allow you to focus
on and share what is good in your world instead of being
depleted by the onslaught of negative messaging.

While setting a boundary may feel as if you are
intentionally excluding experiences or people, it is actually
about establishing limits that allow you to protect your best
interests, as well as those of the loved ones around you.
Boundaries create a healthier environment for our minds
and bodies.

Our earlier example of "Negative Nellie" and her doom-
and-gloom outlook have been scientifically shown to impact

health. Learning how to care about people without taking on their drama, crisis or negativity is one of the masterful ways to set healthy cognitive boundaries.

In her wonderful book, *Boundaries in an Overconnected World*, Anne Katherine simply states,

> "Boundary building can work from outside in or inside out. You can build boundaries with conscious effort and this will change you on the inside – or you can change your insides, and boundaries will automatically form. You can set deliberate limits to protect what you care about – or they will spring up by themselves when you focus your whole self on what matters to you most." (Katherine, 2013, pg.13)

Two simple ways to create healthier boundaries are to learn to say "no" and to simplify your logistics whenever possible. If you find you have trouble saying "no", it might be easier and feel less confrontational to just take a breath and say, "thank you, but that does not work for me". You can reduce the stress of your daily life through stream-lining, by negotiating for something as simple as forming a carpool to work or bicycling to errands. Even having fewer material possessions means less to store, clean and maintain. These are just a couple examples of ways you can afford yourself more time and space to practice Cognitive Replenishment techniques.

Quietude

Quietude is the practice of being still, quiet and present in a nurturing environment, as opposed to withdrawing from external stimuli. It is an opportunity to enjoy your own company, which is a rare and delicious gift.

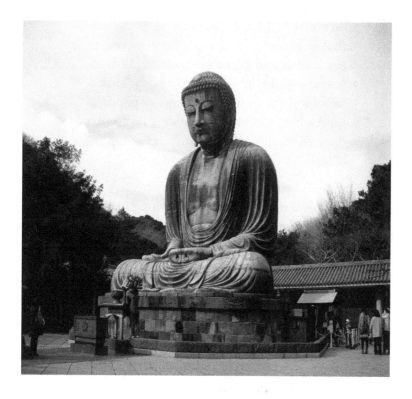

Many great, historical discoveries have occurred when the individual was relaxing and pondering something else. For example, Archimedes' epiphany regarding how to measure the different densities of gold and silver occurred to him while he was relaxing in a bath. Our hero Einstein, was often found daydreaming and watching ribbons of light bounce off the water as he discerned the secrets of the $E=MC^2$.

Quietude serves two purposes. The first is to reduce the elevated cortisol levels from a stressful day. The second is to replenish your mental muscles without having to do a thing.

"Studies done at the Franklin Institute, a
Philadelphia-based science research center,
on stress and the adrenal glands show
that even low-level chronic noise increases
aggression and decreases cooperation and
is associated with increased risk for such
serious physiological problems as peptic
ulcers, high blood pressure, cardiovascular
disease, stroke and even suicide."
(Clores, 2012)

Quiet time helps maintain your sanity. In the Tao Te
Ching, a book of life wisdom from China, this is referred
to as "Wei Wu Wei" (*Doing Not Doing*) and is revered as a
masterful practice.

"Without opening your door, you can open
your heart to the world. Without looking
out your window you can see the essence
to the Tao. The more you know, the less you
understand. The Master arrives without
leaving, sees the light without looking,
achieves without doing a thing."
–*Tao Te Ching*, as translated by Stephen
Mitchell

The "Mind Dump" Technique

When you feel frustrated with a situation or person, breathe
deeply nine-times, grab a pen and paper and prepare to
enjoy a Mind Dump. Write out all the stuff bothering you,
in an uncensored way, so you can let it rip without hurting
anyone. Get it off your chest. Then tear it up, throw it away,

or burn it safely. It has been demonstrated that there are even benefits to those who write out their frustrations in cursive (Klemm, 2013). That's a double whammy – you get to let the steam out of your radiator in a safe manner and stimulate synchronicity between the two hemispheres of your brain (Asherson, 2013).

Employ the Technique of "AND" Thinking

(This is one of my all-time favorites as a *worryholic* in recovery.)

One of the top-ten of success skills. Whenever you feel defeated, hopeless, upset, angry or unsure, allow yourself to gently express your distress, then add *"AND"* followed by a great alternative outcome. An example might be, "Shoot! I missed the bus to work, AND now I get to take a nice, unexpected walk in the sunshine."

"AND" thinking is completing your emotionally charged, worrisome, negative thoughts with what you would prefer. Another example is, "Wow! These clothes do not fit me as well as they once did…AND, now I get to spend some quality time with my best girlfriends going shopping." You see, end on the note of a better outcome. Turn real time lemons into future lemonade. It is like casting a positive vote for yourself and the ultimate outcome. Try it, have fun and be creative! This will help develop your positive imagination as well.

- "AND" I will get to eat ice cream after the tonsillectomy

- "AND" my neighbor enhanced the view after surprisingly taking down that tree

- My friend had to cancel our dinner plans, "AND"

now I have the opportunity to read the last chapters
of that delicious spy novel

It takes a bit of practice to find the silver lining during
a difficult moment, but "AND" thinking is a great way to
reduce stress and remember the positive, as you navigate
this unpredictable and wacky world.

Reminiscing

Remarkably, we can intentionally stimulate our creative
problem solving abilities through reminiscing. A study by a
trio of Harvard researchers found that when groups of
subjects were forced to reminisce about the specific details
of a past experience they were better able to access their

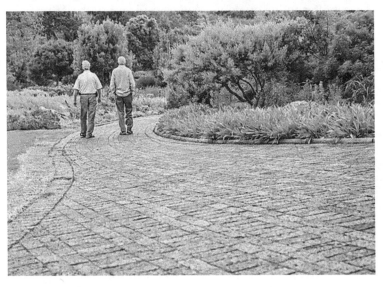

"divergent thinking" or creative problem solving (Madore,
2015). Perhaps this is what Einstein was referring to as a
higher level of thinking. You can provide better quality
solutions to the problems at hand, by taking a walk down
memory lane. Simple, fun and worth the effort.

Practical Optimism, an Affordable and Great Tonic

Besides seemingly having a better time in life, the optimists around you also reap significant health benefits as a result of their upbeat perspective. Optimists are happier and live longer, literally. A longitudinal Mayo Clinic study of 800 people over a thirty-year period showed that pessimists were nineteen-percent more likely to die before their optimistic brethren.

> "A pessimistic explanatory style, as measured by the Optimism-Pessimism scale of the MMPI, is significantly associated with mortality." (Maruta, 2000)

Dr. Martin Seligman, the father of positive psychology says it clearly, "People who make permanent and universal explanations for good events, as well as temporary and specific explanations for bad events, bounce back from troubles briskly and get on a roll easily when they succeed once" (Seligman, 2002).

He has even written a book on the topic of *Learned Optimism*, which is defined as the cultivation of the talent for joy. Learned optimism is at the opposite end of the spectrum from *learned helplessness*. Dr. Seligman posits that consciously challenging any negative self-talk can effectively promote optimism. He currently offers an online test for those interested in assessing their present state of positivity at: http://web.stanford.edu/class/msande271/onlinetools/ LearnedOpt.html

Optimists also possess what is referred to as resilience, the ability to bounce back from life's tragic circumstances. It was discovered that soldiers who possessed a practical type of optimism recovered from extreme wartime trauma without depression or post-traumatic stress disorder

(Charney, 2002). Optimism was also the primary factor that determined whether a veteran was able to recover from the trauma they experienced as a prisoner of war. Altruism, humor and a meaningful life were deemed as secondary factors aiding in their emotional recovery (Charney, 2002).

According to Dr. Charney, a practical optimist can assess their difficult situation in a realistic manner, while seeking a solution that has not yet presented itself. During times of great difficulty, a practical optimist may not know how they will solve the problems at hand, but they are confident a way will appear as they actively pursue a remedy. This type of confidence takes a bit of faith and a lot of positive imagination.

Positive imagination is a skill that can be cultivated. Appreciating the goodness and beauty that exists in your world is a simple first step. Once you acknowledge the good in front of you, it is easier to expand this practice as outlined below.

Here are some suggestions for how to develop a more positive imagination:

- **Situational** – Imagine having a good time with the people you are going to meet today before you see them. As you leave the house imagine you are going to have a great day, or that you will enjoy the time you're going to spend with a loved one, or that you will find a win/win solution at a business meeting. Try to imagine great outcomes before the fact and then see the effects this has on the quality of your interactions.

- **Environmental** – surround yourself with people who are kind, genuine, caring, honest and capable of appreciating your finer qualities. People who believe in goodness and see it in the world.

- **Self-Talk** – Learn to catch and correct the nasty messages each of us inflicts upon ourselves in the guise of motivation. These messages aren't motivating, they are demeaning and often insidious. Affirming the good and learning from our mistakes is the best we can do as humans. Say nice things about yourself and to yourself often. It is worth it. If you're not sure how to, sit with a safe friend and ask for three things they really like about you. Hearing it out loud really helps. Or, begin by telling yourself," I am a lovable being".

Affirmations: Challenging Negative Self-talk

When you are ready to challenge negative self-talk, achieve new goals, or intentionally own the good that already exists in your life, try affirmations.

Affirmations are a potent way to generate uplifting energy when life gets tough. Affirmations are best performed with pen on paper. This method stimulates your brain and working memory more comprehensively (Asherson, 2013). A legal pad sits in my house ready to capture both affirmations and my quarterly mind dump.

At the Vast Institute, we work with many folks to learn the benefit of affirmations on Cognitive Replenishment. When you take ten-minutes to challenge the beliefs that promote low self-esteem, you begin to take charge of the quality of the messages you present to your mind. We want to stimulate your positive imagination on purpose. In these moments craft a supportive, positive statement to countermand the negative one in your head. This is where your "AND" thinking will pay off big time. Let's say I missed a baseball practice or class play because I forgot to look at my notebook during an overwhelming day. I might feel stupid, silly and embarrassed. This is the perfect time to start with a basic affirmation like:

"I am lovable even when I make mistakes."

Make sure to write it out in the first, second and third person, five times for each. Insert your name as well.

For example:

"I, Michelle, am lovable even when I make a mistake." x 5

"You, Michelle, are lovable even when you make a mistake." x 5

"She, Michelle, is lovable even when she makes a mistake." x 5

Have fun with it. Feel free to change the words to match who you are. I find that my affirmations have evolved to be easier and kinder after years of practice. As you write esteem-boosting thoughts down, a voice may arise to dispute your positive claim. That is your Ego protecting you from change, in case the change could be harmful to you. Just breathe through your "Negative Nellie" thoughts and continue to write out your statement of support for forty-days. This timeframe anchors the positive idea into your cognitive realm. Enthusiastically saying your affirmations out loud with gusto into the mirror awards you extra credit.

Gratitude

Gratitude not only appeals to our higher minds, it also enhances our well-being. It is a virtue that can actually improve the quality of our lives. Studies have shown a distinct connection between a state of thankfulness and a person's well-being. Thus, something as simple as giving thanks benefits everyone (Sasone, 2010).

Some of the physical health benefits of gratitude include a boost to the immune system, as well as a reduction in stress levels. Furthermore, grateful people tend to be more optimistic and better at coping with the stress in their lives. They also tend to take better care of themselves through habits like a healthy diet and regular exercise (Heubeck, 2006).

Cultivating gratitude can help people reframe their perspective and experiences in a positive way, helping them to feel that their life is manageable and meaningful (Lambert et al, 2009). As we stated earlier, personal coherence is vital in achieving Cognitive Replenishment. The Heart Math Institute says one of the emotional states that elicit personal coherence is gratitude.

So take a moment out of your day to give thanks for the good that already exists in your life. Be grateful for a warm shower, a good meal, a child who is healthy, a wonderful vacation, quality time with family, a vibrant mind, people who care, a clean bed, jam from strawberries, mint chocolate chip ice cream, etc. If you celebrate the small things the big ones can more easily find you.

Celebrate Your Heroes, Large and Small

Make an effort to acknowledge the accomplishments large or small of those you deem to be inspiring - your heroes. It could be: Grandma for raising and feeding eight amazing kids; the PTA director who makes sure that parents and teachers work together; CEO Elon Musk, who generously gifted his solar wall patents as open source, so that anyone can access and improve on Tesla's technologies. Or, as we previously mentioned, people like Mr. Craft and Commander Cernan, who risked their lives to expand the grasp of all humankind. Take time to notice other people's contributions to your life and the overall good of the world. Once you start looking for examples they seem to multiply. This is all about where you choose to pay attention.

Braincations

Spending time with nature is the original, most cost effective, stress reduction technique and healing force available. Making time to experience or simply imagine nature is called a Braincation. It is a great way to combat cognitive fatigue and replenish your mental muscle. Braincations are one way to positively balance corporate overload. Cognitive science is just beginning to fathom the positive impact nature has on us, and the findings are impressive.

- **Increased attention span.** Nature restores our ability to focus. In a 2008 study by University of Michigan psychologists, Berman, Jonides and Kaplan, they found that directed attention and the ability to concentrate on a task were improved by walking outside or even just looking at photos of nature.

- **Better memory.** The same study reported a twenty-percent improvement in recalling a series of numbers after one hour of interacting with nature. In later research, Berman showed that participants who walked through an arboretum in the cold of winter performed better on cognitive testing than they had before the walk and outperformed subjects who took their walk through an urban setting (Berman, 2012).

- **Reduced stress.** An earlier study at the University of Michigan (1989) revealed that a view of trees and flowers at work promoted lower stress levels, higher job satisfaction and fewer physical ailments in employees as compared to their co-workers, who could only view other buildings from their desk.

- **Improved mood.** It has been shown that following a stressful event, workers who viewed scenes of water or trees were able to recapture a positive mood more quickly than those who viewed urban scenes. Living in rural settings can support your mental health. City dwellers are twenty-percent more likely to develop anxiety disorders and forty-percent more likely to develop other mood disorders compared to people living in rural settings (Ellison, 2015). These findings offer further evidence of the value of Braincations.

- **Greater creativity.** By spending four days in the back country students participating in an Outward Bound course enhanced frontal lobe activity by forty-percent. Increased frontal lobe activity has been linked to greater creativity (Atchley, 2012).

All of these studies support the idea that there is a tremendous benefit to be derived from exposure to nature. Urban planners have been mandated to take this into consideration as they design the cities of our future. Spending time viewing or being in nature provides intentional mental refreshment, especially for children.

> "Contact with nature helps children to develop cognitive, emotional and behavioral connections to their nearby social and biophysical environments. Nature experiences are important for encouraging imagination and creativity, cognitive and intellectual development and social relationships."
> (University of Washington Department of Urban Forestry & Urban Greening Research)

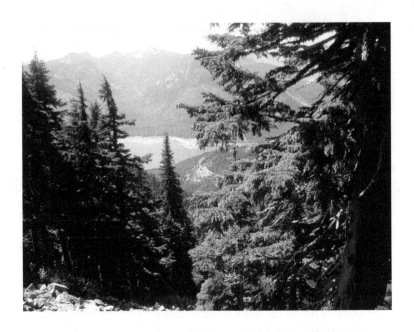

So go ahead and shamelessly enjoy nature. Stare happily at trees, birds, waves, clouds, flowers and all the beautiful things that you pass by each and every day. Awe can be an emotional trigger for the experience of personal coherence.

> "Those who contemplate the beauty of
> the earth find reserves of strength that
> will endure as long as life lasts. There is
> something infinitely healing in the repeated
> refrains of nature - the assurance that dawn
> comes after night, and spring after winter."
>
> – Rachel Carson, *Silent Spring*

There you have it, a VAST menu of techniques designed to enhance a Cognitive Replenishment practice and fertilize the soil of your positive imagination. This toolkit includes: enjoying that good belly laugh, remembering the good old days, or spending time in various ways communing with nature. These methods are free and simple to implement, so choose the one that suits you best each day. Experiment with these techniques whether they are familiar or brand new to you while you feel good. This will allow you to identify which ones provide that mental lift when you need it most.

To aid with your Cognitive Replenishment practice VAST has provided five items of ongoing support.

1. The eighteen individual tools outlined in this chapter that can make a huge difference in the quality of your cognitive and emotional life when implemented.

2. The Cognitive Replenishment Practice Journal found in Appendix A. This tool provides feedback as to which techniques work best for you in different circumstances. For example, if you cannot leave your desk for a break, perhaps listening to birdsongs for three-minutes will refresh you. At other times, a mind dump can help release some of the outrage you feel in a safe, non-threatening way. When you are completely stuck, roll-out that Duchene grin in the bathroom mirror and instantly gather your confidence back.

3. The VAST Institute® Braincation Enjoyment Service. This yearly subscription provides replenishing images and videos of nature. Visit www.vastinstitute.com to subscribe today and restore your brain chemistry to its full vibrancy. This photo and video collection from the VAST Archives will replenish you personally, while supporting the VAST mission to imagine that human kindness prevails.

4. Glossary with definitions of terms used in this book can be found in Appendix C.

5. The VAST Cognitive Replenishment Bibliography for further reading and research can be found in Appendix D.

When all else fails you can always laugh at the situation. As Norman Cousins' amazing recovery indicated, being amused by life can lighten the hardest moments in a healing manner.

> "Mirth is like a flash of lightning that breaks through a gloom of clouds and glitter for the moment. Cheerfulness keeps up daylight in the mind, filling it with steady and perpetual serenity."
>
> — Samuel Johnson

So claim your mirth, your healthiest mind and begin to experience Cognitive Replenishment with us now.

CHAPTER SEVEN
REVIEW QUESTIONS TO CONSIDER:

1. What unconventional method helped to heal Norman Cousins?

2. Name two characteristics of emotionally intelligent people.

3. What type of smile brightens up your brain chemistry?

4. Name one benefit of being an optimist.

5. Name three of your favorite cognitive replenishment mind moves.

CHAPTER EIGHT

Coaxing the Milk of Human Kindness to Flow throughout the World

I choose to imagine the milk of human kindness flowing throughout the world. That is what *my* positive imagination chooses to visualize. If that thought feels good to you too, we can share this meme. You can also imagine your own wonderful and exuberant scenario, whatever feels exquisite to you!

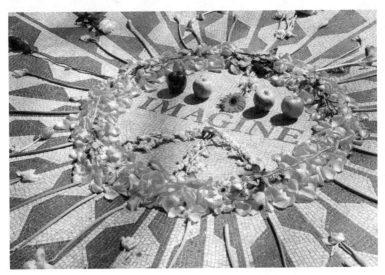

At the VAST Institute, we strongly believe that if we can imagine something we can assuredly work together to create it. As one begins to refresh their cognitive realm, they will be able to access divergent thinking. Refreshing your cognitive realm using our techniques allows you to tap into positive imagination, creating a better life while working in harmony to create a better world.

"When I first met Michelle, I was unhappy, confused and uncertain about most aspects of my life... I was living my life in a very reactive state and had no personal authority or true consciousness about myself and actions. I have grown and evolved considerably...and I have to thank Michelle for guiding me along the way... My relationships with my family and friends have all developed and improved. My confidence and sense of worth have increased tenfold. When I reflect back upon who I was before I started working with Michelle, I feel that I am a different person today. I am very proud of the work that I have done and who I am now." – S.I.

Take a moment each day to tap into the emotions of gratitude, awe, forgiveness and connection. These emotions optimize your biochemical balance so that you experience personal coherence. Allow these moments of positivity to play a vital role in achieving emotional and physical well-being.

When we began this Cognitive Replenishment journey we stated that our goal at the VAST Institute is to offer a simple set of tools to mentally recharge your life. We wholeheartedly believe that you can significantly enhance your quality of life by finding daily, fun ways to:

- Nourish your mind
- Develop a positive imagination
- Take command of where you focus your attention
- Set healthier boundaries

This book was crafted to demystify these four processes and offer up a toolkit to help you launch.

In summary, taking the time to practice Cognitive Replenishment will benefit you by:

- Promoting divergent thinking to create original solutions that suit your values and life.

- Interrupting the cortisol surge that interferes with your ability to tap into your positive imagination.

- Identifying the external and internal factors that can help or hinder your sense of well-being.

- Kick-starting the practice of personal coherence.

- Stimulating significant aspects of emotional resilience during times of extreme stress.

- Becoming aware of and minimizing the FUD resulting from negative messages that distract you from more nourishing ideas.

- Creating a resilient approach that allows you to bounce back from life's traumatic or dramatic moments.

- Allowing you to be your best self when solving difficult and demanding problems at work, home or play.

When we began this journey into the replenishment of your dear mind, Albert pointed out the benefits of developing a positive imagination - it helps us become divergent thinkers and elevates our level of individual and collective problem solving.

There are a multitude of techniques throughout this VAST Institute primer that you can begin utilizing today.

Here are some practical examples to get you started.

- Imagine feeling healthier
- Notice the good in the people around you
- Notice the beauty in your world
- Take daily Braincations
- Take a walk outside in the sunshine and listen for the birds
- Question FUD and the negative assumptions of others
- Surround yourself with kind, appreciative, positive people
- Be gentle and kind with loved ones, including yourself
- Allow yourself the luxury of a good night's sleep (or naps!)
- Love and embrace yourself as a unique gift
- Treat *every* fellow human being with respect
- Establish healthy boundaries
- Imagine peace is imminent
- Imagine a balanced, caring world

CHAPTER EIGHT
REVIEW QUESTIONS TO CONSIDER:

1. Which emotions optimize your personal coherence?

2. Name two benefits you will gain from a cognitive replenishment practice.

3. Name three VAST techniques to kick-start your cognitive replenishment practice.

4. Visualize and describe in detail something outrageously wonderful using your positive imagination. Make sure to engage with all five senses and immerse yourself in the experience for at least three minutes.

NOTES AND INSIGHTS

CHAPTER NINE
Final Thoughts

It is now time for you to get going on those new mind moves!

In reading this book you have begun to imagine a replenished mind - you have begun to kindle your flame. Try different techniques to see what happens.

Let me give you a real life example of how utilizing a combination of VAST Cognitive Replenishment techniques literally saved a client from an unhappy ending. For you see, what you imagine is often limited to what you think is possible, but what you think is possible can be expanded. Like Albert said, imagination is more important than knowledge. A Cognitive Replenishment practice can show you how to be open to possibilities that are currently beyond your imagination.

I once had a client who received fifty-percent of a cash-based business as part of her divorce settlement. The business wasn't doing that well and as her success coach I was tasked with helping her develop and implement a better strategy.

One problem that we faced was that the partner who owned the other fifty-percent of the company lacked confidence in my client's abilities. He kept reassuring her that profitability was always just around the corner, but implied that perhaps she was not up to the task of properly managing and growing the business. He wouldn't come out and say it directly, but he spread F.U.D. by subtly undermining her authority, dismissing her legitimate concerns and setting the blame for the company's lackluster results squarely on her shoulders.

After working with her for about three months to create a roadmap for the business, I noticed a couple things. One, my client had excellent business instincts and was a dedicated leader; the mediocre results of her company did not seem at all to be the result of her poor management. Two, after reviewing the numbers and procedures in great detail, I strongly suspected that someone in the company was embezzling funds, and that this was most likely the cause of the lack of profits. Based on my extensive experience with small businesses, it didn't add up that such a popular establishment that attracted so many customers was just breaking even.

There were a lot of cognitive depletors harming my client in this situation, including the F.U.D. her partner was spreading, the chronic stress she was experiencing, the confusion about why she wasn't making money when she should be, the lack of work-life-balance and the all-consuming effort of saving herself from bankruptcy.

Once my client got over the shock at the possibility that someone she trusted was stealing from her, we set about to discover if our suspicions were correct. Unfortunately they were proven true when we caught her business partner on camera helping himself to a bagful of quarters every night, which did not look like very much, but ended up totaling approximately sixty-thousand-dollars a year. The mystery of the disappearing profits was finally solved.

We gave her embezzling partner, with the support of law enforcement, an ultimatum: either he hand over his half of the business or go to jail. He chose to relinquish his half. We had managed to get rid of the toxic partner, but my client was still faced with a looming bankruptcy. Things were looking bleak and she was feeling hopeless.

This is when I told my client that she in fact had another choice - bankruptcy was not a foregone conclusion. I imagined for both of us that we could sell the business, pay off her debts and at least break-even. I was able to enlist my positive imagination on her behalf, envisioning that it was indeed possible to find someone who would be interested in purchasing this business, and that we could do so with full disclosure, transparency and integrity. Despite all the setbacks it had suffered, it was a great business opportunity for the right person. My client had nothing to lose, and if my optimism did not pan out she could always declare bankruptcy after all.

With our new found optimism, I assessed the business's value with and without the embezzled funds. During this time investors from the east coast contacted us about purchasing my client's company. After many rounds of negotiations we succeeded in selling her company for the full amount that it was worth, even after we disclosed the embezzlement details in their entirety.

This outcome was miraculous for my client. She went from assuming she was going bankrupt to paying off all her debts and even having money left over to seed a new venture. This story dramatically illustrates what can be accomplished with a positive imagination even during the most difficult of circumstances. In the end my client succeeded far beyond what she originally imagined was possible.

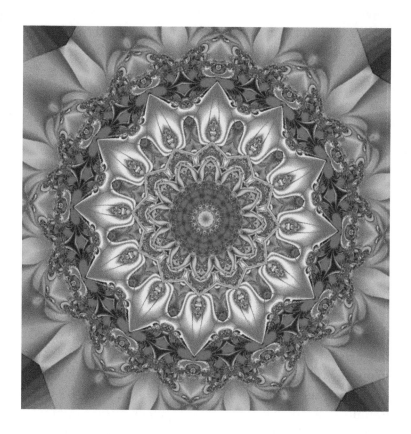

Now it is your turn.

Take your beautiful, healthy, respectable mind back from the bombardment of incessant negative messaging. I am personally working on this one myself, with vigor and dedication. I do this because I know that in healing my mind and treating it well, I can begin to imagine a world of beauty, peace and sufficiency. Once imagined, we can collectively move mountains or conquer impossible dreams. That is the secret that Commander Cernan and Mr. Kraft shared with me. Watch what unfolds with a bit of positive imagination on your side. Albert Einstein once confided to a colleague that positive imagination was his lifelong friend.

"When I examine myself and my method of thought, I come close to the conclusion that the gift of imagination has meant more to me than my talent for absolute knowledge." (Calaprice, 2011, pg. 26)

Thank you for wanting to be a happier, healthier human being. Each time one of us sees the greater good it makes it easier for all of us to move in a saner, more cooperative direction. The millions of choices we make each day to develop our best self, promotes coherence and harmony. Each time we contribute our unique gifts to the Cognitive Replenishment of the collective imagination of the human family, we grow as the self-respecting inhabitants of this blue-jeweled planet.

Go forth, and in the company of your dearest friends, family and community, imagine a wonderful world into existence. The Vast Institute will here be doing the same in our own caring and dedicated manner. As we kindle our own flame and inspire others to do the same, we strive to illuminate the path before us and together create a brighter future. We will imagine that peace be with you and yours now and in all ways. Thank you.

If you would enjoy VAST support in developing your Cognitive Replenishment Practice, please join our VAST Institute® Cognitive Replenishment teleconference at www.vastinstitute.com.

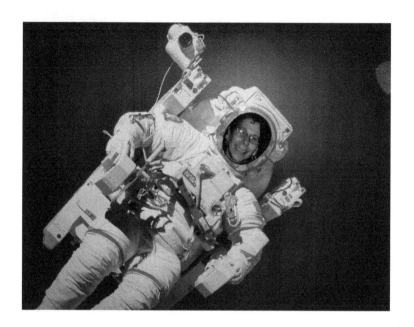

CHAPTER NINE
REVIEW QUESTIONS TO CONSIDER:

1. How can FUD negatively impact your work environment?

2. Name one strategy that promotes positive outcomes?

3. What role can positive people play in helping you achieve success?

4. Michelle's positive imagination was so powerful it propelled her into space! What amazing things will your positive imagination make possible?

ACKNOWLEDGEMENTS

I would like to share a heartfelt note of deep appreciation to the many talented and caring colleagues, friends and clients whose kindness and generosity continue to encourage, inspire and awe me. Without their encouragement and hard work this jewel of a book would still reside in the realm of my imagination.

I especially want to thank:

- Mike Ament, for countless efforts, priceless contributions, patient wrangling and for believing that the VAST Institute and its sparkle do indeed matter.

- Dr. Lori Adcock, for your patience and dedication to making this book as scientifically accurate as possible, as well as accessible to all readers.

- Clara Lawryniuk, for your word craft, editorial wisdom and articulate gifts. I have become a better writer and communicator because of your insightful guidance.

- Kim Whitson, for your fine-toothed comb review, your love and perspective.

- Jonathan Van Valin for work on organizing earliest drafts.

- Catherine Corley, for your enthusiasm, depth of understanding and grace.

- Cynthia Chomos, your forward-thinking suggestions, beauty and optimism.

- Sergey Vesmanov, for for your friendship, pedagogical input and VAST support.

- Anne Bean, for your design magic and ensuring that this book would visually delight our audience.

- Deb LaRoche, for your ongoing encouragement, support of our most innovative endeavors, and generous heart.

- Betts Ashcraft, for your bravery.

- The Hartman family, for their ongoing enthusiasm for the VAST mission.

- Barbara Standiford, for your light-laden support.

- Dr. Friedemann Schaub, for your example, gifts and caring.

- Commander Eugene Cernan, for your inspiring heroism.

- Christopher C. Kraft, Jr., for your faith that we could get the job done.

- Our VAST network of friends, clients and colleagues for their magnificence.

- Albert Einstein, for your expansive imagination.

- Anamaria Lloyd, for igniting the quest for a wonderful title.

And, to all the kindhearted souls in the world who make this planet a more loving place every day in a 100-zillion different ways.

Thank you,

Michelle Sherman

West Seattle, WA, 2017.

Appendix - A

VAST INSTITUTE®
COGNITIVE REPLENISHMENT
PRACTICE JOURNAL

Dear Fellow Human Being,

Pick and choose the Cognitive Replenishment techniques that work best for you. Experiment with them. Small changes, done with enthusiasm, can bring about great results. Review chapter seven and eight for fan favorites such as:

- Braincations
- Laughter
- Time with true friends
- "AND" thinking
- Optimistic moments
- Music of the nourishing kind
- Sitting with pets
- Cuddling with a sweet person
- Breathing in the scent of flowers in the air
- Watching the clouds roll by as they create beautiful patterns
- Meditating
- Feeling grateful for what you already have
- Smiling from a warm place in your heart

Day:_____

Cognitive Replenishment choice:_____

Gift of it:_____

Notes and insights: _____

_____

_____

Day:_____

Cognitive Replenishment choice:_____

Gift of it:_____

Notes and insights: _____

_____

_____

Day:_____

Cognitive Replenishment choice:_____

Gift of it:_____

Notes and insights: _____

_____

_____

Day: _____

Cognitive Replenishment choice:_____

Gift of it: _____

Notes and insights: _____

_____

_____

Day: _____

Cognitive Replenishment choice:_____

Gift of it: _____

Notes and insights: _____

_____

_____

Day: _____

Cognitive Replenishment choice:_____

Gift of it: _____

Notes and insights: _____

_____

_____

Day:_____

Cognitive Replenishment choice:_____

Gift of it:_____

Notes and insights: _____

_____

_____

Day:_____

Cognitive Replenishment choice:_____

Gift of it:_____

Notes and insights: _____

_____

_____

Day:_____

Cognitive Replenishment choice:_____

Gift of it:_____

Notes and insights: _____

_____

_____

Day: _____

Cognitive Replenishment choice: _____

Gift of it: _____

Notes and insights: _____

_____

_____

Day: _____

Cognitive Replenishment choice: _____

Gift of it: _____

Notes and insights: _____

_____

_____

Day: _____

Cognitive Replenishment choice: _____

Gift of it: _____

Notes and insights: _____

_____

_____

Appendix - B

VAST INSTITUTE®
ANSWER KEY FOR
CHAPTER QUESTIONS

CHAPTER ONE

1. What does the *plenish* in cognitive replenishment mean?
To fill up, stock or furnish.

2. Name two cognitive replenishment techniques.
Exhibiting a positive imagination or considering practical optimism.

3. What is the opposite of cognitive replenishment?
Cognitive depletion.

4. Why is developing a positive imagination worthwhile?
Your imagination provides the placeholder for a brighter future until that future can actually occur.

5. Name two benefits you stand to gain from a cognitive replenishment practice.
Less stress. Greater ease and enjoyment of life.

CHAPTER TWO

1. What does Albert think is more important than knowledge?
Imagination.

2. **Name one reason people often lack a positive imagination.**
   They are surrounded by Negative Nellies, or are mentally exhausted.

3. **Name one quality Highly Sensitive People (HSP) possess.**
   Intuition, or social awareness.

CHAPTER THREE

1. **Name two reasons why Negative Nellies often commands your attention.**
   You brain is wired to intentionally emphasizes bad news, commanding your attention. We have mirror neurons that allow for emotional contagion from negative people in our life.

2. **List three ways negative messages arrive on your doorstep.**
   Newspapers, sad stories from neighbors, reality TV drama.

3. **What is the Hawthorne effect?**
   An observer will unintentionally become part of the experiment and influences its results. Your presence impacts the outcome of the experiment. You make a difference.

4. **What can happen when you experience an amygdala hijack?**
   An amygdala hijack focuses our attention on problems instead of the solutions.

CHAPTER FOUR

1. **What does cognitive replenishment fuel?**
   Our positive imagination.

2. **What feelings indicate an experience of personal coherence?**
   When we experience being in the flow of life and everything seems to be working smoothly. We feel satisfied and content.

3. **What has contributed to our boldest successes as a species?**
   The unwavering positive imagination of a multitude of diverse people working together (i.e. synergy).

4. **What did the NASA team focus its attention on and how did that enable us to reach to the moon?**
   By focusing on the desired outcome and having faith in its possibility, rather than focusing on the challenges and seeming impossibility.

CHAPTER FIVE

1. **Name the fab four of happy brain chemicals (aka DOSE)?**
   Dopamine, Oxytocin, Serotonin & Endorphin.

2. **What is the connection between mirror neurons and emotional contagion?**
   Mirror neurons help us to experience the emotional states of others, which allows for emotional contagion to occur.

3. **What occurs when oxytocin interacts with estrogen?**
   This chemical interaction enhances the collaborative impulse.

4. **What is a meme?**
   A meme is a unit for carrying cultural ideas, symbols, or practices that can be transmitted from one mind to another through writing, speech, social media, gestures, rituals, or other imitable phenomena.

5. **Name two outcomes of chronic stress.**
   Elevated cortisol levels, which can lead to lowered immunity and an increase in inflammation. Other outcomes include: an increase in fat deposits in abdominal organs, decrease in muscle mass, elevated blood sugar levels and impaired cognitive function.

CHAPTER SIX

1. **What does FUD stand for?**
   Fear, Uncertainty & Doubt.

2. **Name three ways to enhance your sense of wellbeing.**
   Nourish your mind. Develop and apply a positive imagination. Take command of where you place your attention.

3. **Name two cognitive depletors that you have experienced.**

   i. _____

   ii. _____

4. **Why is it important to set cognitive boundaries?**
   We need cognitive boundaries to allow our minds and bodies to rest and refresh. They are a way to protect ourselves from cognitive depletion.

CHAPTER SEVEN

1. **What unconventional method helped to heal Norman Cousins autoimmune illness?**
   Laughter.

2. **Name two characteristics of emotionally intelligent people.**
   Recognize emotions in others. Handle their relationships in a socially competent manner.

3. **What type of smile brightens up your brain chemistry?**
   A Duchenne smile.

4. **Name one benefit of being an optimist.**
   Optimists possess what is referred to as resilience, the ability to bounce back from life's tragic circumstances.

5. **Name three of your favorite cognitive replenishment mind moves.**
   i. _____

   ii. _____

   iii. _____

CHAPTER EIGHT

1. **Which emotions optimize your personal coherence?**
   Gratitude, awe, forgiveness and connection.

2. **Name two benefits you will gain from a cognitive replenishment practice.**
   Helping identify the external and internal factors that can further or hinder your sense of well-being. Allowing you to be your best self when solving difficult and demanding problems at work, home or play.

3. **Name three VAST techniques to kick-start your cognitive replenishment practice.**
   Notice the good in the people around you. Take a walk outside in the sunshine. Establish healthy boundaries.

4. **Visualize and describe in detail something outrageously wonderful using your positive imagination. Make sure to engage with all five senses and immerse yourself in the experience for at least three minutes. Write down your vision to help anchor the experience.**

CHAPTER NINE

1. **How can FUD negatively impact your work environment?**
   By undermining authority, dismissing legitimate concerns and spreading blame and doubt about competent people.

2. **Name one strategy that promotes positive outcomes?**
   Positive imagination, or divergent thinking.

3. **What role can positive people play in helping you achieve success?**
   They can help you to imagine positive outcomes and design positive strategies when you are cognitively depleted.

4. **Michelle's positive imagination was so powerful it propelled her into space! What amazing things will your positive imagination make possible?**

Appendix - C

GLOSSARY & ADDITIONAL RESOURCE MATERIAL

Boundary Violation: "A boundary violation is an action (or failure to act) that weakens or breaks a boundary, harming the entity inside it. There are two types of violations...an intrusion violation penetrates the entity, creating breach or interruption....a gap violation is created when one fails to act or respond when an action is called for." (Katherine, 2013, pg. 23)

Braintrust: An advisory board, cabinet, council, etc.

Catecholamine: "Any of a class of aromatic amines that includes a number of neurotransmitters such as epinephrine and dopamine." — Oxford Dictionary

Cognitive Realm: the VAST Institute cognitive realm includes, but is not limited to 1) where you invest your attention 2) your level of consciousness (as exampled by Dr. David Hawkins map of consciousness in Power versus Force, pg. 69) and 3) your self-talk.

Cognitive Replenishment: the intentional care and nourishment of one's mind, through the practice of self-care, positive imagination and appropriate boundaries, that results in greater creativity and innovative outcomes.

Cognitive Replenishment Practice:

1. Become aware of and expand the experience of personal coherence, diminish the drama in your world.
2. Learn to set cognitive boundaries that are healthiest for you! See the beauty.
3. Practice your favorite Cognitive Replenishment techniques and see progress.
4. Develop the ability to return to a relaxed state after life's usual stressors.
5. Access your higher problem solving powers to fuel your positive imagination, unleash original thinking and create a quality of life that is presently beyond your imagination.

Cognitive Depletors: that which discourages or drains your mental energy, neural chemical balance, stamina or optimism. Something that causes cognitive depletion.

Divergent Thinking: Imaginative thinking, characterized by the generation of multiple possible solutions to a problem, often associated with creativity. The concept was introduced in 1946 by the US psychologist Joy Paul Guilford (1897-1987)"— Oxford Reference Dictionary. At VAST we refer to Divergent thinking as Original Thinking.

Duchenne smile: involves contraction of both the zygomatic major muscle (which raises the corners of the mouth) and the orbicularis oculi muscle (which raises the cheeks and forms crow's feet around the eyes).

Emotional Contagion: the tendency to feel and express emotions similar to and influenced by those of others; also, the phenomenon of one person's negative thoughts or anxiety affecting another's mood.

Episodic Memory: is the memory of autobiographical events (times, places, associated emotions, and other contextual who, what, when, where, why knowledge) that can be explicitly stated. It is the collection of past personal experiences that occurred at a particular time and place. They allow you to figuratively travel back in time to remember the event that took place at that particular time and place.

FUD: the low level vibes of fear, uncertainty and doubt that are often used to exploit or manipulate your actions to benefit others.

Hawthorne effect: (also referred to as the **observer effect**) is a type of reactivity, which individuals modify or improve an aspect of their behavior in response to their awareness of being observed.

Learned Optimism: the idea in positive psychology that a talent for joy, like any other, can be cultivated. It is contrasted with learned helplessness. Learning optimism is done by consciously challenging any negative self-talk.

Negative Nellie: a person who can find the fear, uncertainty and doubt in every situation and who's willing to share it with anyone who'll listen.

Original Thinking: the creation of new thought forms to stimulate grander outcomes.

Personal, Group and Community Coherence: according to the Heart Math Institute, Coherence is the harmonious flow of information, cooperation, and order among the subsystems of a larger system that allows for the emergence of more complex functions. This higher-order cooperation among the physical subsystems such as the heart, brain, glands, and organs as well as between the cognitive, emotional, and physical systems is an important aspect of what we call coherence. – From a monograph from HeartMath Institute (2003) authored by Rollin McCraty, PhD, which is entitled *Physiological Coherence.*

Positive Psychology: a relatively new branch of psychology, which focuses on how to help people prosper and experience happier, healthier lives.

Practical Optimist: A kindhearted and positive person, who believes in goodness, that their choices make a difference and that positive outcomes are possible.

Prefrontal Cortex: "The most typical psychological term for functions carried out by the prefrontal cortex area is executive function. Executive function relates to abilities to differentiate among conflicting thoughts, determine good and bad, better and best, same and different, future consequences of current activities, working toward a defined goal, prediction of outcomes, expectation based on actions, and social "control" (the ability to suppress urges that, if not suppressed, could lead to socially unacceptable outcomes)."-Wikipedia

Synergy: the cooperation of two or more individuals that produces a combined effect that is greater than the sum of their separate effects.

Worryholic: someone with a tendency to ruminate on the myriad of things that could possibly go wrong in a manner that is detrimental to their personal coherence.

Additional Resources for Support

- American Board of Psychologists: www.abpp.org
- Adult Children of Alcoholics:
  www.adultchildren.org
- Adult Children of Dysfunctional Families:
  www.adultchildrenofdysfunctionalfamilies.com
- Al anon meeting groups: www.al-anon.org
- www.thefearandanxietysolution.com
- VAST Institute® Braincation subscription

Appendix - D

BIBLIOGRAPHY

Allred K.D., Byers J.F., Sole M.L. (2010). The effect of music on postoperative pain and anxiety. *Pain Manage Nurse.* 2010 Mar;11(1):15-25.

Aron, Elaine N., Ph.D. (1996). *The Highly Sensitive Person: How to Thrive When the World Overwhelms You.* Broadway Books, New York.

Asherson, Suzanne Baruch (2013). The Benefits of Cursive Go Beyond Writing. *The New York Times*, New York.

Atchley, RA, Strayer DL, Atchley P. (2012). *Creativity in the wild: improving creative reasoning through immersion in natural settings*, NIH.

Barbero G.J., Shaheen, E. (1967). Environmental failure to thrive: A clinical view; *J Peds* 71(5):639-644

Bauchner H. et al. (2007). Failure to Thrive. In: Kliegman RM, Behrman RE, Jenson HB, Stanton BF, eds. *Nelson Textbook of Pediatrics.* 18th ed. Philadelphia Pa: Saunders Elsevier; 2007:chap 37

Berk, Lee (1989).Neuroendocrine and Stress Hormone Changes During Mirthful Laughter, *American Journal of the Medical Sciences*: December, 1989.

Berkowitz, Gale (2002). *UCLA Study On Friendship Among Women: An alternative to fight or flight.*

Berman, Jonides & Kaplan (2008). The Cognitive Benefits of Interacting With Nature. *Psychological Science.*

Berman, M.G., Kross E., Krpan K.M., Askren M.K., Burson A., Deldin P.J., Kaplan S., Sherdell L., Gotlib I.H., Jonides J. (2012). Interacting with Nature Improves Cognition and Affect for individuals with Depression. *Journal of Affective Disorders,* Epub 2012 Mar 31

Black, O.H. and Garbutt, L.D. (2002). Stress, Inflammation and Cardiovascular Disease, *Journal of Psychosomatic Research,* Vol 52, Issue 1 p. 1-23, January 2002.

Bloom, William (2001). *The Endorphin Effect.* Little Brown Book Group, London.

Cadzow, R.B. and TJ Servoss (2009). The association between perceived social support and health among patients at a free urban clinic. *Journal of the National Medical Association.* 2009. 101: 243-250.

Cain, Susan (2012). *Quiet: The Power of Introverts in a World That Can't Stop Talking.* Crown Publishers, New York.

Calaprice, Alice. (Ed.). (2011). *The Ultimate Quotable Einstein.* Princeton, N. J.: Princeton University Press.

Campanini P., Conway P.M., Neri L., Punzi S., Camerino D., Costa G. (2013). *Workplace bullying and sickness absenteeis.* Epidemiol Prev., 2013 Jan-Feb;37(1):8-16.

Carnegie, Dale (1990). *Stop Worrying and Start Living.* Mass Market Paperbacks.

Carson, Rachel (1962). *Silent Spring.* Houghton Mifflin Company, NY 1962.

Charney, Dennis, M.D. Ehrenkranz Anne, Ehrenkranz Joel, (2005). *The Psychobiology of Resilience to Extreme Stress:*

Implications for the Prevention and Treatment of Mood and Anxiety Disorders.

Clores, Suzanne (2012). *The Benefits of Quiet for Body, Mind and Spirit.* Next Avenue / Twin Cities Public Television. 2015.

Cousins, Norman (1979). *Anatomy of an Illness as Perceived by the Patient,* WW Norton and Company.

de Niet G., Tiemens B., Lendemeijer B., Hutschemaekers G. (2009). *Music-assisted relaxation to improve sleep quality: meta-analysis.* J Adv Nurs. 2009 Jul;65(7):1356-64.

Ellison, Marc (2015). *Hiking in Nature = Improved Mental Health?.* Hiking Research, October 2015.

Eng, P.M. et al. (2002). *Social ties and change in social ties in relation to subsequent total and cause-specific mortality and coronary heart disease incidence in men.* American Journal of Epidemiology, 155: 700-709.

Goleman, Daniel (1997). *Emotional Intelligence: Why it can Matter More than IQ.* Bantam Books.

Goleman, Daniel (2007). *Social Intelligence - The Revolutionary New Science of Human Relationships.* Bantam Books.

Harlow, Harry (1958). *The Nature of Love.* American Psychologist, 13, 673-685.

Hawkins, David R. (1995). *Power versus Force: The Hidden Determinants of Human Behavior.* Hay House, Inc.

Heuback, Elizabeth & Louise Chang, MD, (2006). *Boost Your Health With a Dose of Gratitude.* Web MD.

Heuback, Elizabeth (2007). *Violent Images Impact Kids Differently.* Web MD.

Iacoboni, Marco (2008). *Mirroring People: The New Science of*

How We Connect with Others, Picador, NY.

Katherine, Anne M.A. (1991). *Boundaries: Where You End and I Begin*. Simon & Schuster.

Katherine, Anne (2013). *Boundaries in an Overconnected World: setting limits to preserve your focus, privacy, relationships and sanity*, New World Library.

Klemm, Willliam, Ph.D (2013). *Biological and Psychology Benefits of Learning Cursive: don't let your schools stop teaching cursive*, Psychology Today.

Kraft T.L., Pressman S.D. (2012). *Grin and bear it: the influence of manipulated facial expression on the stress response*, Psychological Science, Epub.

Lambert, Nathaniel M., Steven M. Grahamb, Frank D. Finchama and Tyler F. Stillmana (2009). *A changed perspective: How gratitude can affect sense of coherence through positive reframing*. The Journal of Positive. Psychology, Vol. 4, No. 6, November 2009, 461–470.

Landau, Elizabeth (2013). This is your brain on music. CNN.com.

Lin S.T., Yang P., Lai C.Y., Su Y.Y., Yeh Y.C., Huang M.F., Chen C.C. (2011). Mental health implications of music: insight from neuroscientific and clinical studies. *Harvard Review of Psychiatry*. 2011 Jan-Feb;19(1):34-46.

Madore, Addis, and Schacter (2015). The Key to Creativity is in Imagining the Details, *Journal of Psychological Science*.

Martin, William (2000). *The Sage's Tao te Ching*.

Maruta, Cooligan, Malinchoc, Offord (2000). Optimists vs Pessimists: Survival Rate Among Medical Patients Over a 30-Year Period, *Mayo Clinic Proceedings*,

Volume 75, Issue 2, February 2000, Pages 133-134

Mayo Clinic Staff (2013). *Chronic Stress Puts Your Health at Risk.* The Mayo Clinic, July 2013.

McCraty, Rolllin, PhD (2003). *Physiological Coherence*, HeartMath Institute Monograph.

McCutcheon-Rosegg, Susan & Erick Ingraham (1984). *Natural Childbirth the Bradley Way.*

Mitchell, Stephen (1988). *Tao Te Ching.* Harper & Row, Publishers, Inc. New York.

Naime, Gary, PhD (2014). *WBI US Workplace Bullying Survey.* Workplace Bullying Institute.

Nagasawa, Miho (2009). *Hormones and Behavior*, Azabu University.

Nagasawa, Miho (2015). Oxytocin-Gaze Positive Loop and the Co- Evolution of Human – Dog Bonds. *AAAS Science*, vol 348, no 6232, p 333-336.

Rauh, Sherry and Louise Chang, MD (2011). Video Game Addiction No Fun. *Web MD Archives.*

Reblin, M. and B.N. Uchino (2008). Social and emotional support and its implications for health. *Current Opinion in Psychiatry.* 2008. 21: 201-205.

Redd, WH et al (1994). Fragrance administration to reduce anxiety during MR imaging. *Journal of Magnetic Resonance Imaging.* 1994. Jul-Aug: 4(4):623-6

Sansone, Randy A., MD & Lori A. Sansone, MD, (2010). Gratitude and Well Being: The Benefits of Appreciation. *Psychiatry* (Nov. 2010): Vol. 7, No. 11, pp. 18-22.

Schaub, Friedemann (2012). *The Fear and Anxiety Solution: A Breakthrough Process for Healing and Empowerment with Your Subconscious Mind,* Sounds True Inc., Boulder CO.

Selhub, Eva, M.D., Logan, Alan C. N.D. (2012). *Your Brain on Nature: The Science of Nature's Influence on Your Health, Happiness and Vitality,* Wiley Press.

Seligman, Martin E.P., Ph.D. (2002). *Authentic Happiness: using the new positive psychology to realize your potential for lasting fulfillment,* Free Press.

Seligman, Martin E.P., Ph.D. (1990). *Learned Optimism,* Pocket Books, Simon and Schuster, NY.

Scott, Elizabeth M.S. (2011). Cortisol and Stress: How to Stay Healthy- Cortisol and Your Body. *About.com Guide,* September 22, 2011 reviewed by the Medical Review Board.

Smith, K. Annabelle (2013). A WWII Propaganda Campaign Popularized the Myth That Carrrots Help You See in the Dark. Smithsonian.com.

Stamatakis, E. (2011). Screen-based entertainment time, all-cause mortality, and cardiovascular events: Population-based study with ongoing mortality and hospital events follow-up. *Journal of the American College of Cardiology,* 57(3), 292-299.

Taylor, S. E., Klein, L.C., Lewis, B. P., Grunewald, T. L., Gurung, R. A. R., & Updegraff, J. A. Behavioral Responses to Stress: Tend and Befriend, Not Fight or Flight , *Psychol Rev,* 107(3):41-429.

Waitley, Denis Ph.D. (2010). *The Psychology of Winning.* www.waitley.com.

Wegner and Pennebaker (1992). *Handbook of Mental Control.*

Weinschenk Susan Ph.D. (2014). Texting addiction - Are You Addicted to Texting? Or why you can't ignore your smartphone, *Brain Wise.*

Weinstein, N. (2009). Can nature make us more caring? Effects of immersion in nature on intrinsic aspirations and generosity. *Personality and Social Psychology Bulletin,* 35, 1315.

Woolston Chris (2015). Health Benefits of Friendship, *Emotional Health Library.*

Yager, Jan PhD (2002). *When Friendship Hurts: How To Deal With Friends Who Betray, Abandon, Or Wound You.* Touchstone.

Young, Kimberly PsyD, Clinical Director of the Center for On-Line Addiction (2011). Caught in the Net: How to Recognize the Signs of Internet Addiction - and a Winning Strategy for Recovery, *WebMD.*

Zillmann, Dolf (1979). *Hostility and Aggression.* Hillsdale NJ, Lawrence Erlbaum Associates, Publishers.